Self Assessment in Paediatric Musculoskeletal Trauma X-rays

Full the full range of M&K Publishing books please visit our website:
www.mkupdate.co.uk

Self Assessment in

Paediatric Musculoskeletal Trauma X-rays

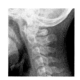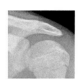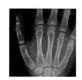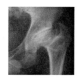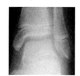

Karen Sakthivel-Wainford

H.D.C.R (R), PGCert, MSc
Advanced Radiographer Practitioner, Leeds General Infirmary, UK

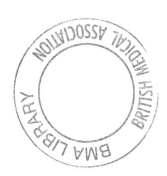

Self Assessment in Paediatric Musculoskeletal Trauma X-rays
2nd edition

Karen Sakthivel-Wainford

ISBN: 9781910451-07-6

First published 2008. This revised edition 2016

British Library Catalogue in Publication Data
A catalogue record for this book is available from the British Library

Notice
Clinical practice and medical knowledge constantly evolve. Standard safety precautions must be followed, but, as knowledge is broadened by research, changes in practice, treatment and drug therapy may become necessary or appropriate. Readers must check the most current product information provided by the manufacturer of each drug to be administered and verify the dosages and correct administration, as well as contraindications. It is the responsibility of the practitioner, utilising the experience and knowledge of the patient, to determine dosages and the best treatment for each individual patient. Any brands mentioned in this book are as examples only and are not endorsed by the Publisher. Neither the Publisher nor the author assume any liability for any injury and/or damage to persons or property arising from this publication.

The Publisher
To contact M&K Publishing write to:
M&K Update Ltd · The Old Bakery · St. John's Street
Keswick · Cumbria CA12 5AS
Tel: 01768 773030 · Fax: 01768 781099
publishing@mkupdate.co.uk
www.mkupdate.co.uk

Designed & typeset by Mary Blood
Printed in England by McKanes Printers, Keswick

Contents

Acknowledgements

Firstly to Dr Arthur, consultant paediatric radiologist, for the sharing of her knowledge and enthusiasm, which imparted to me an interest in paediatric trauma. Also for her continued support during her time at the Leeds Trust. I wish her a happy retirement.

To the radiology departments of Leeds General Infirmary and Wharfedale General Hospital, for their continued support and for the use of their radiographs in this book. Thanks also to the many radiographers and radiographer practitioners at Leeds General Infirmary, who keep bringing to my attention interesting and useful cases, for this book and my teaching.

Lastly, this book is in memory of my husband's grandmother, who helped me adjust to Indian village life.

Also thanks to my husband, who has not only supported me, but is my computer expert when everything goes wrong!

Introduction

Many nurse practitioners and radiographer practitioners view paediatric trauma radiographs with a certain amount of trepidation. Rightly so – paediatric radiographs can be difficult to interpret, requiring additional learning (additional courses), and experience, but that is the challenge and interest of paediatric trauma.

Children, infants and adolescents are not like 'little adults' with regard to trauma, as we shall discuss in Chapter 2. This book, like the previous edition, is written specifically for radiographers, nurse practitioners and radiographer practitioners. It is meant to represent sitting in on a reporting session with a radiologist or reporting radiographer, where you are asked to write a report or comment, but also asked several questions. The book is intended to support whatever course you are attending, or to encourage you to go on that 'paediatric course'.

It starts with a chapter on non-accidental injury (NAI) from different perspectives: that of a nurse practitioner, Louise Lindsay, with an interest in paediatrics; Joyce M. Clayton, a social worker specialising in children; and Emily Hargreaves, a paediatric team leader, who discusses the skeletal survey. This highlights the pathway a child suspected of NAI may take, from initial presentation and the Emergency Nurse Practitioner's suspicion, to involving social services, to the skeletal survey.

This is followed by a brief description of the different types of paediatric fractures that may occur, with examples of these in the following cases. The next chapter looks at the pathway for the limping child and the role x-ray plays in this.

As in the previous edition, a series of cases on paediatric trauma follows, on which you are asked to write reports and provisional image evaluations, as well as sometimes answering a few questions.

I have concentrated on the areas of paediatric trauma that are most commonly presented to an emergency department or minor injuries unit; hence there are more cases of foot and ankle, wrist and hand, and elbow, as these are the most frequent attendees. These are also the areas that radiographer practitioners and nurse practitioners are most likely to be reviewing. There are some new cases in this second edition, especially in areas that people find difficult to interpret, such as the elbow, and those areas that commonly present at an emergency department or minor injuries unit.

There are eight sections in total: trauma radiographs of the wrist and hand (20 cases); elbow and forearm (15 cases); shoulder (10 cases); foot and ankle (20 cases); knee (10 cases); hip and pelvis (10 cases); the rest of the axial skeleton (10 cases); and finally a section with mixed paediatric trauma cases, for you to test yourself further. This last mixed section now includes 25 cases. The cases have all been anonymised, hence there are no names and sometimes no anatomical markers. This also sometimes results in some of the radiographic anatomy not being present. Each case has some appropriate clinical history with it, but this is often not the original clinical history in order for the patient to remain anonymous.

Lastly there is a list of texts and journals I have found particularly useful in researching paediatric trauma. As for whether all the cases have trauma demonstrated on the radiograph or not, that is for you to decide.

1.

Non-accidental injury

Introduction

Non-accidental injury is thought to have been first described by Caffey in 1946. While he was reviewing children with subdural haematomas, he found that many of these children also had other fractures that were at different stages of healing. Most cases of non-accidental injury are brought to medical attention in children younger than 18 months; whereas most trauma in children tends to occur after 18 months of age, when they are more physically active.

There are several identified risk factors for NAI:

● Premature baby, or serious neonatal illness
● Disabled child
● Failure to bond
● Fretful, crying child
● Young, immature or inexperienced parents
● Social deprivation
● Drug or alcohol abuse
● Lack of good parenting models.

However NAI can occur in any child. The classic radiographic signs of NAI, or 'battered child syndrome' as Caffey first called it, are:

● Multiple fractures at various stages of healing
● Rib fractures.

Metaphyseal injuries are often occult, the most common sites being the knees and ankles. Metaphyseal injuries are rare due to other trauma in children under two years of age. If an arm or a leg is continuously shaken, twisted or grabbed, the loosely attached periosteum along the diaphysis will rise. (There are fewer Sharpey's fibres in this age group; see Chapter 2). This will result in subperiosteal bleeding, and a periosteal reaction will be seen – normally one week after the trauma. Periosteal reaction is non-specific for NAI and can have many causes, including infection. However, metaphyseal fractures are said by some authors to be pathognomic of NAI and are present in 39–50 per cent of cases (Knipe & Bhattacharya). The periosteum is tightly attached to the metaphysis; and shaking or twisting of limbs results in a fracture of the metaphysis (the so-called bucket handle or corner fracture). However, pathology can also cause metaphyseal injuries.

An interesting article by Wheeler and Hobbs (1988) reviewed cases referred to the child abuse team over 10 years in Leeds, from 1976 to 1986, and found that 50 children referred with suspected NAI were found to have conditions that mimicked NAI. These included nine children with impetigo, five with blue spots, five with haemostatic disorders, eight with bone disorders, and one who had evidence of NAI as well as a condition mimicking abuse. This demonstrates what a difficult diagnosis NAI is for all involved. Radiographically, two of the most common pitfalls in diagnosing NAI are skeletal dysplasia and metabolic conditions.

Diaphyseal fractures are the most common NAI injury and they are highly suspicious in non-ambulant patients. Transverse fractures are less suspicious than spiral or oblique fractures, but care should be taken not to confuse a 'toddler's fracture' with NAI (see Chapter 3).

In children younger than two years of age, NAI is the foremost cause of serious head injury involving skull fractures. Falls from a height of less than 1.25 metres are unlikely to result in serious head injury. If, at initial presentation, the clinician is suspicious that a skull fracture is due to NAI, then (in accordance with NICE guidelines January 2014) the patient should have a CT scan within 1 hour (see Chapter 10, Case 86).

Rib fractures are rarely the result of an accident, as ribs are extremely plastic and elastic (see Chapter 2) and therefore difficult to fracture. Rib fractures from NAI are often multiple, bilateral and posterior. Rib fracture are clinically and radiographically occult but thought to occur in up to 25 per cent of cases, hence the follow up chest x-ray after a skeletal survey, to increase the chance of viewing occult rib fractures.

Knipe and Bhattacharya comment that radiologists are often the first to suspect NAI when confronted with particular injury patterns; and a knowledge of these is essential if the opportunity to prevent further harm to the child is not to be missed. In my opinion, all professionals involved with the child have a responsibility to be alert to the possibility of NAI. At the same time it is essential that suspicion is not raised inappropriately, as the consequences for innocent parents or guardians are significant. Some important questions to consider are:

- Do the clinical details fit the injury?
- Was there a delay in presentation?
- How does the child interact with the parents or guardians?

The radiologist has an important role in reviewing the skeletal survey. The ability to date injuries is critical for medicolegal purposes and this must be done carefully; there are many specialist texts that offer specific guidance on this.

- In general, traumatic periosteal injury can be seen for up to 7 days after injury and can therefore be used for dating.
- Diaphyseal injuries start healing at 1 week. Healing should be complete by 12 weeks.
- Metaphyseal injuries do not heal with periosteal reaction, and if visible they are less than 4 weeks old.

Everyone plays an important role in identifying and documenting NAI. The rest of this chapter looks at NAI from the perspectives of three groups of professionals, and follows the path a child may take when presenting to A&E, from being reviewed by the Emergency Nurse Practitioner (ENP), to the involvement of the social worker, to the skeletal survey that is carried out by radiographers after the child has been placed in a place of safety.

The Nurse Practitioner's perspective

Louise Lindsay
RN, ENP Sister

This section covers the role of the Emergency Nurse Practitioner (ENP) in the care of children with non-accidental injuries (NAIs) and will cover some of the laws and legislation surrounding this issue, clinical signs to look out for and what the ENP needs to do if he or she suspects NAI. There are many issues within child protection and I propose to deal with the key points the ENP should be aware of.

Every week in England and Wales at least one child dies following cruelty (National Society for the Prevention of Cruelty to Children, 2004). The people most likely to die a violent death are babies under one year who are four times more likely to be killed than the average person (Youd, 2005). However, abuse can occur at any age in a child's life, in any culture and within any social background and environment. Therefore ENPs need to be vigilant to the possibility of NAI for all children attending a minor injuries unit (MIU). All ENPs must be familiar with and follow legislation and their organisation's procedures, policies and protocols for safeguarding and promoting the welfare of children in their area and know who to contact in their organisation to express concerns about a child's welfare. This can be very complex and therefore daunting for any healthcare professional as they have to gain a clear understanding of what the implications and impacts are so that they can include these in their working practices. Ultimately, the ENP is accountable and responsible legally and professionally to themselves, to the patients, for the safeguarding and welfare of the child and its family, and to the employing institution and the nursing profession. The Government issued a non-statutory guidance booklet in 2006 on 'What to do if you're worried a child is being abused' (Department of Health, 2006a). This is very helpful for understanding and working within the requirements of the Children Act 1989 and 2004.

So, what does safeguarding and promoting the welfare of children mean? The Children Act, (p. 8, 3.1) gives the following definition:

- protecting children from maltreatment
- preventing impairment of children's health or development
- ensuring that children are growing up in circumstances consistent with the provision of safe and effective care, and
- undertaking that role so as to enable those children to have optimum life chances and to enter adulthood successfully.

The Children's Act 1989/2004 offers the most comprehensive legislative framework with regard to the rights, care and protection of children and the responsibilities of those who care for them. There are other laws and legislation and each geographical NHS area is responsible for developing their own procedures following that legal framework. The procedures for the area in which I work are detailed by the Leeds Local Safeguarding Children Board (LSCB) in the Inter-Agency Child Protection Procedures. It is now a mandatory requirement that all ENPs achieve the Level 1 Child Protection E-Learning Module (2006) produced by the Child Protection Health Advisory Group, Trustwide Child Protection Steering Group and the Leeds Named Nurses: Child Protection Group which covers all relevant areas of child protection. All ENPs should be aware of the West Yorkshire Safeguarding Procedures which can be accessed from www.leedslscb.org.uk.

Also the Children Safeguarding Nursing Team within Leeds Teaching Hospitals NHS Trust (LTHT) produced a supporting Paediatric Liaison Resource File. This is easy to follow and contains the *Framework for the Assessment of Children and their Families* (DOH, 2000) which is an essential tool for the ENP to use when working towards safeguarding and promoting child welfare (see Figure 1.1). Any one of the three domains in the triangle within the Framework may raise an issue about a child. The Resource File also lists all the healthcare professionals, their areas of responsibility, names and telephone numbers, together with flowcharts of actions to take when concerned about a presenting child or their family. It is also the ENP's responsibility to keep up to date with all changes as they arise by research, reading and attending relevant courses and by liaising appropriately with other healthcare professionals. ENPs should work within the Assessment Framework. If an ENP suspects non-accidental injury, he or she must follow all protocols, policies, procedures and guidelines on child protection set out by their organisation.

Armed with all the above, the ENP needs to be able to identify an NAI. There are many definitions of child abuse. Abuse and neglect are forms of maltreatment of a child. Somebody may abuse or neglect a child by inflicting harm, or by failing to act to prevent harm. Children may be abused in a family or in an institutional or community setting by those known to them or, more rarely, by a stranger. They may be abused by an adult or adults, or another child or children (HM Government, 2006b, p. 37, 1.29).

As soon as a child and family attend the MIU it is the responsibility of all the multi-disciplinary team to pass on all observations and information to the ENP. Any information could be vital for the ENP's assessment and safeguarding of the child. The ENP may be the first professional a child and family come into contact with.

Youd (2005) asserted that all emergency nurses, not only those working in traditional emergency departments but also and particularly those with new autonomous roles in walk-in centres, MIUs, children centres and primary care environments, may be the only professionals seeing particular children during care episodes (p. 15). She also states 'front line emergency nurses must ensure they have the necessary core skills, knowledge and competencies in assessing and treating children' (p. 16).

Figure 1.1 **Factors affecting child welfare**

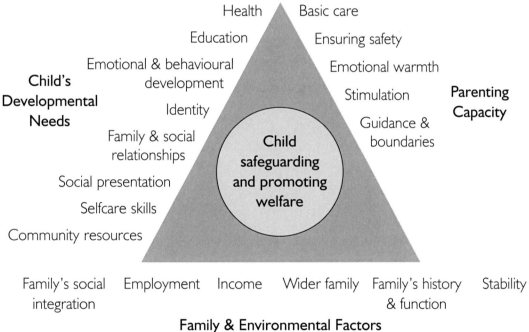

The ENP should start the clinical assessment by interacting professionally, positively and in a friendly manner using good communication skills in an effort to put the child and family at ease. The ENP should communicate with the child in a way that is appropriate to their age, understanding and preference. Whaley and Wong (1991) indicate that knowledge of development theory will enable the nurse to choose words that are appropriate for the child's chronological age and anticipated understanding. The skill involved is not only using the correct words but also interpreting verbal and non-verbal feedback from the child. Morgan (1991) states that using the correct approach to an injured child will help in gaining the child's co-operation and trust. The ENP also needs to gain the trust of the family. Dolan (1997) reminds us that no child can be thought of in isolation from their family. The assessment includes obtaining the history of the presenting complaint, i.e. which part of the body, what has happened, when, how and where it was witnessed. Throughout the assessment the ENP should monitor the following:

- interactions and reactions of the child with the family, looking for any odd behaviour
- compatibility of the history with the developmental stage of the child
- how the child looks and whether there are signs of failure to thrive
- whether the mechanism of the injury fits with the history and injury
- whether there has been a delay in attending the MIU for treatment
- whether there is a history of previous attendances at the MIU or main site A & E departments
- what the child says about the accident
- whether the account is vague or lacking in detail
- whether the parent's and child's accounts of the injury are the same
- whether staff members within the MIU have been given different accounts of what happened; this is why it is vital the multidisciplinary team shares information.

This approach is supported by Wynne (1994) who states that the presentation of history may give clues or raise the question of abuse.

None of the above is foolproof and there can be many other factors that may come to the ENP's attention during the assessment. If there are previous attendances, the ENP needs to know what these were for and documentation about previous attendances should be reviewed. Also, the ENP must take into account multiple previous attendances to MIUs and emergency departments as these could show a pattern of abuse.

The ENP then carries out a thorough clinical examination of the child, in accordance with local guidelines, whilst being aware of the common sites for NAIs. It is of great value during the examination if the ENP, with the help of other colleagues and involving the family, can use distraction techniques with the child. According to Gay (1992) distraction, relaxation, imagery and reinforcement are all effective ways of reducing stress in children undergoing procedures. In all cases the ENP should identify any bruises of varying ages and colours, swellings, wounds, deformities, bony tenderness or any abnormalities. It is important for the ENP always to observe the child's reactions to the clinical examination and to look for any signs of neglect, other injuries or other concerns. If the ENP observes a failure to thrive or has other concerns then they should weigh the child and chart this using the centile chart creating a base record for future reference. Greenidge (1997) believes the knowledge of the related anatomy and physiology is vital to ensure an accurate, systematic and holistic assessment. The ENP should gain an impression of the type of injury and decide on the next plan for the child. This could be requesting an x-ray before decision making, referring to the main hospital site or other healthcare professionals for further assessment, or on-site diagnosis, treating and discharging. If the ENP decides an x-ray is required, this has to be carried out in accordance with their organisation's policy for referral of patients to radiology, also taking into account their local guidelines and protocols, and must not go out of these boundaries. The ENP should stay within their Code of Conduct and Scope of Professional Practice (UKCC, 1992a, 1992b). If the area for x-ray is not within the ENP's protocol this must be referred to a main hospital site for an A & E doctor to review. If a child has been x-rayed on site, the ENP must make a clinical decision based upon the radiograph and clinical findings and then follow this up with the appropriate action. For the ENP to interpret and report on x-rays they must have the appropriate training and authorisation and, if not, the x-ray must be reported on by a radiographer or authorised colleague. Should an NAI be suspected, then the ENP should begin to document concerns and follow documented procedures. In the first instance, this could be liaising with school nurses, health visitors, GPs and other healthcare professionals by telephone, to ascertain if the family have a social worker, any previous history of problems or if the child is subject to a child protection plan. A list of children who are subject to a child protection plan is accessible from Children and Family Social Care. This is managed by Safeguarding Children Senior Co-ordinators (LSCB, 2007). These general enquiries can give the ENP valuable information before any approach is made to the family or any further action is taken.

Wynne (1994) states that staff working in this difficult field must be trained and supported. The work is skilled, time consuming and emotionally taxing. The consequences for the child and family if the abuse is not recognised or is wrongly diagnosed are considerable.

ENPs should bear in mind that a referral for a child could result in access to services under Section 17 of the Children Act 1989 for family support before the situation deteriorates to a level where the child must be referred for protection under Section 47 of the Act. If unsure, the ENP should always liaise with the Children Safeguarding Nursing Team. If the x-ray interpretation of a suspicious fracture indicates that this could be an NAI, this must be reported to the Children Safeguarding Nursing Team and Children and Young People's Social Care.

After gathering all the information, if a cause for concern with Child Protection issues exists, this falls under Section 47 of the Children Act 1989/2004 (Child Protection). The objective of local authority enquiries conducted under Section 47 is to determine whether action is needed to promote and safeguard the welfare of the child or children who are the subject of enquiries. In the great majority of cases children remain with families and, even if concerns about abuse or neglect are substantiated, enquiries should be conducted in a way that allows for constructive relationships with families (LSCB, 2007).

At this point, the ENP must relate their professional concerns to parents and carers and be prepared to answer questions openly and honestly, unless to do so would affect the safety and welfare of the child. If an ENP wishes to refer to Children and Young People's Social Care because it is felt a child is at risk then it is good practice to always seek the consent of the parent to make that referral, unless to do so would put the child at risk. If the ENP feels a child is at risk of significant harm they do not require the consent of the parent to refer. Likewise, if the child is already subject to a child protection plan there is no need to gain consent. In *Working Together to Safeguard Children* (Department of Health, 1999, p. 40, para 5.6), it states 'while professionals should seek, in general to discuss any concerns with the family and, where possible, seek their agreement to making a referral to social services, this should only be done where such discussion and agreement-seeking will not place a child at increased risk'. The powers, duties and roles of agencies involved, and their own legal rights, should be explained to the parents. Care should always be taken if the ENP is aware of a situation with the child and/or family which could become volatile and he or she should not put themselves in a vulnerable position.

If the ENP is aware that a social carer is already involved with the family then they should be informed of the cause for concern during office hours or to the Emergency Duty Team (EDT) outside office hours. If there is no previous social care involvement the ENP should contact the duty social care team on the call centre number during office hours. This should be documented and the ENP should keep a copy for their own records and fax a copy to the appropriate professionals and agencies who require the information. The ENP should also indicate whether they have informed the child and/or parents of the referral and whether the child and/or parents have indicated their agreement to information about them being shared between agencies for the purposes of assessment.

The individual ENP continues to be responsible for raising their concerns and communicating with health visitors, school nurses, the Children Safeguarding Nursing Team and Young People's Social Care, EDT social carers and the police. They should make all the referrals themselves and not assume that these will be done by someone else; otherwise there is a risk of breakdown in communication and a child could become at risk. It is best practice to carry out all these referrals within 24–48 hours.

The child must be referred by the ENP to medical staff within their organisation at the main hospital's emergency department. It is good practice and necessary for the ENP to liaise verbally with a senior A&E doctor, senior paediatric registrar and any other specialist doctor as appropriate, together with the paediatric area. Also the ENP should ensure the Children Safeguarding Nursing Team are made aware. Again this communication is essential for safeguarding the welfare of the child.

It is crucial that all assessments, examinations, clinical findings, descriptions and drawings of injuries are documented and the appropriate proformas are used in all cases.

Comprehensive, accurate and timely documentation is necessary for high-quality healthcare (Cooper, 2000).

The Trustwide *Child Protection Policy* (Child Protection Health Advisory Group, 2006, p.43) states that accurate record keeping is an essential element which must underpin child protection work. ENPs must remember that the function of accurate record keeping is not only to enhance seamless care but is also evidentially crucial. The Policy also states that effective child protection work relies not only on excellent interagency communication but also on the quality of recorded information. It not only clarifies the nature, extent and the development of concerns but also helps to identify patterns of behaviour. In addition, it states that basic principles of record keeping must be adhered to and must be contemporaneous in nature, e.g. entries must be legible, written in black ink, signed with name printed beneath signature, dated and timed. Also any record of the child's words should be verbatim and not an interpretation of what the child meant. If the ENP asks the child questions, these should be included in the record also.

Once everything has been completed, the ENP arranges for the safe and secure transportation of the child or family to the main hospital emergency department. This is a crucial point to prevent further risk or harm to the child. If the child is suspected to have suffered abuse this may involve organising an ambulance. If abuse is confirmed the police may already be involved and safe transport or transfer is mandatory in these cases.

The ENP may be the first professional the child and family come into contact with and therefore plays a crucial role in identifying suspected safeguarding issues or abuse or NAIs in the first instance. This can be very challenging, complex and time consuming but also very valuable and rewarding. The ENP has a frontline role in protecting the child and preventing further risk or harm. Within my own area of work all staff are constantly vigilant, sharing information and highlighting to each other any concerns or anomalies which may arise with the presenting child or family. This multidisciplinary team effort is of great value and importance and should be occurring in all work environments that provide services for children. Is this happening in your workplace? In addition, the legislation, procedures, policies and protocols are available to support ENPs and multidisciplinary teams in their work and they should consult their own safeguarding policy and procedures for further guidance. Added to this, with the efficient child protection networks that exist there is no excuse not to be effective in the child protection process. This effectiveness could prevent the further harm or future death of a child.

Working Together to Safeguard Children states that 'safeguarding and promoting welfare of children – and in particular protecting them from significant harm – depends on effective joint working between agencies and professionals that have different roles and expertise' (Department of Health, 2006b, p. 33, 1.14). Junior and senior staff have different roles in safeguarding individual children. 'Individual children, especially some of the most vulnerable children and those at greater risk of social exclusion, will need co-ordinated help from healthcare professionals' (1.14). 'In order to achieve this joint working, there need to be constructive relationships between individual workers, promoted and supported by all' (1.15). We should all work together to safeguard and protect the child's welfare and there should always be partnership with families and colleagues throughout the care process.

The Social Worker's perspective

Joyce M. Clayton

Regional Paediatric Specialist Social Worker, Certificate of Qualification in Social Work (CQSW), practice teacher.

Paediatric x-ray interpretation is a crucial part of dealing with a non-accidental injury. This x-ray is evidence and gives feedback to the paediatric consultant who can then review their medical and social information and decide within a strategy discussion with Social Care and other relevant agencies whether this is indeed a non-accidental injury.

The role of social workers in non-accidental injuries is a particularly difficult one. It has been made more difficult by attitudes of some parts of the media. It seems that in some people's opinion social workers cannot do right; they either fail to protect children from injury, or when they act to prevent a child being injured they are accused of wrecking families' lives and have been described as 'do-gooders' and 'interfering busybodies'.

The national agenda

Since 2003 the Government has been outlining its *Every Child Matters* agenda. This develops a new approach for delivering services to children, young people and families. It will radically change the way we work together, from teachers and social workers to voluntary organisations and primary care trusts.

The Government published its *Every Child Matters* green paper in 2003 as a response to Lord Laming's inquiry into the death of Victoria Climbié. He identified poor integration and communication between services and a lack of accountability as serious failings that contributed to the death of Victoria.

A wide range of national legislation and guidance now informs *Every Child Matters*, including:

- The Children Act 2004
- The National Service Framework for Children, Young People and Maternity Services
- The Five-Year Education Strategy
- The Childcare Strategy
- Choosing Health
- Youth Matters.

The Leeds Safeguarding Board consists of the following membership:

- Leeds City Council Social Care Department
- Leeds City-wide Health Services
- Leeds Mental Health Services NHS Trust
- Education Leeds
- Leeds City Council Department of Legal Services
- Leeds City Council Neighbourhood and Housing Services
- Leeds City Council Department of Leisure Services
- Leeds City Council Early Years Service
- West Yorkshire Police
- West Yorkshire Probation Service
- NSPCC (National Society for the Prevention of Cruelty to Children)
- Voluntary agencies
- Leeds Inter-Agency Project Women and Violence
- CAFCASS (Children and Family Court Advisory Support Service)
- Youth Offending
- Connexions West Yorkshire
- HM Wetherby young offenders unit.

The above agencies play an essential part in the process of protection of children. The work of the statutory and voluntary agencies is co-ordinated by the Leeds Safeguarding Board. The agencies meet regularly to review existing policies and services, and monitor child protection activity in the city.

Levels of intervention model for safeguarding children and young people

In order to offer a framework for child protection work, the following model provides a tool for identifying clearly the purpose of any interventions.

- **Preventative:** Work that aims to minimise the risks of children being abused or abusing other people both now and in the future, including work with families under pressure or stress.
- **Protective:** Work that aims to protect children from abuse when concerns have been identified, including enabling children to protect themselves where possible and seek support if and when they need to. It includes developing understanding, skills, information and child protection procedures that aim to protect children from abuse, and providing access to family support.
- **Supportive:** Work that aims to support children who have experienced any form of abuse, aiming to meet their needs, support the process of recovery, minimise the possibility of abuse occurring again or it contributing to learnt behaviours.

A case study

I will explain the process of child protection and investigating a non-accidental injury using an anonymous family. The presenting family are mother Anna aged 25 years, father Robert aged 29 years and baby Tony aged 5 months, the couple's first child. Tony's parents are married and therefore both have parental responsibility for him according to the law.

Anna has brought baby Tony to the emergency department screaming. She herself is distressed and crying. Staff have great difficulty ascertaining what has happened because of the distress of both mother and child. This is complicated because Anna cannot speak or understand English. Robert follows and is angry that Anna has brought baby Tony to the hospital. He is so angry staff have called security to calm the situation so that Tony can be medically examined. Robert is requested to calm himself or the police will be called. He is told that his threatening behaviour to his wife and intimidating attitude to the staff will not be tolerated. He is oblivious to the fact that his pattern of behaviour is emotionally damaging to babies, children and young people, primarily to his own son and others waiting in the accident and emergency department. On presentation to hospital there often is anger and frustration but the child's well-being and protection is paramount. There should always be respect for culture, class, disability, illness and religion to safeguard the child's welfare.

At this point it is urgent for an interpreter to be sought to be present during baby Tony's medical or, if that is not possible, a telephone link. During the interpreted discussion and examination the consultant ascertains that Anna has been at work and Robert was babysitting. Robert informs the doctor and nurse that baby Tony rolled off his parents' bed onto the carpeted floor. He was screaming when Robert picked him up and put him in his cot. He was still screaming in his cot when his mother Anna returned from work. Robert was downstairs drinking heavily and watching television. Anna picked up their son and ran to the hospital. On examination the doctor suspects a fractured femur. He requests an x-ray and the outcome is a spiral fracture of baby Tony's femur. This injury is serious and in my experience can be caused by a forceful pulling, twisting action. A skeletal survey would follow to check that there are no other fractures, new or old and healed. Baby Tony is admitted to the children's orthopaediac ward to have his leg put in traction. As his parents are agreeing to his admission he is now in a 'safe place' whilst information is gathered and an enquiry commenced.

The nursing sister contacts the social care office and asks if the family are known. Past computer records inform that baby Tony has already had a bruise on his forehead at age four months. The explanation was accepted as it was feasible. However at that time Anna had gone into a women's hostel for a week after a domestic argument that was attended by the police. She was observed there to be a caring mother who was attached to her baby son. She returned to Robert after he had pleaded to give him another chance. As the explanation for the fracture is not compatible with the father's story of a fall from the bed, there now needs to be further investigation to protect baby Tony.

The next process is a strategy meeting, usually held at the hospital. The duty team manager chairs and records the minutes of the meeting. The agencies involved need to be coordinated from health, education, police, social care, the voluntary sector and youth justice services if appropriate. This process is a shared responsibility needing accurate information that is non-judgemental. It is not just Social Care's responsibility to safeguard children and young people.

If a baby, child or young person is brought to the accident and emergency department of the hospital with an injury and there is no matching explanation for that injury then it is in the child's best interests that a Section 47 enquiry commences. This action places a duty on the following:

- local authority
- local education authority
- housing authority
- health authority, strategic health authority or National Health Service trust
- the person authorised by the Secretary of State; they are to help an authority with its enquiries in cases where there is reasonable cause to suspect that a child is suffering, or is likely to suffer, significant harm.

As professionals we are all working together to safeguard children. They all deserve the opportunity to achieve their full potential. This is set out in the five outcomes within the *Every Child Matters Children and Young People's Plan*, and are as follows:

- to stay safe
- to be healthy
- to enjoy and achieve
- to make a positive contribution
- to achieve economic well-being.

Becoming a parent or carer (with parental responsibility) does not mean that there is a perfect way to bring up children. Good parenting involves caring for children and providing them with basic needs. This means giving children love and warmth, keeping them safe and providing them with stimulation needed for their development. This then assists them to meet their potential within their capabilities. This is equivalent to a stable home environment where parents and carers give consistent appropriate guidance and boundaries.

Babies, young children and adolescents are more challenging than they ever have been. Parents and carers need support and empowerment within that role. As professionals we should acknowledge that parents asking for help is a positive step and not a sign of failure, which is how many feel when they need support.

As in the Children Act 1989 and 2004, a child is anyone who has not yet reached their eighteenth birthday. 'Child' therefore means 'young person'. The fact that a young person has reached the age of sixteen years, living independently or in foster care, in the armed forces, prison or a young offenders' institution, does not change his or her status or entitlement to services or protection under the Children Act of 1989.

A child or young person being brought to the accident and emergency department will initially be seen by the triage nurse. The information gathered at this stage has to be accurate and recorded. If the explanation by the parent or carer does not satisfactorily match the injury then the social care department should be contacted. In the city of Leeds, this would be the Hospital Team during office hours for the hospitals and, outside of office hours, the Emergency Duty Team. This referral should be a rapid response for the child's safety and a written referral highlighting the concerns should follow and also a medical report.

In good practice, baby Tony's parents should be informed and have a discussion regarding this decision. There is often anger and frustration at this time but the child's well-being and protection are paramount, during and after the enquiry. Being honest with parents and giving them feedback after each stage is crucial in working alongside the family and ultimately the child or young person. Respecting culture, class, disability, illness and religion is all part of safeguarding the child's welfare.

At the strategy meeting, the accident and emergency staff may have only just met the family; however the school, family doctor, and health visitor may have known the family for years and can bring crucial background information to assist the discussion. This information is unknown at presentation at the hospital.

After the strategy meeting the family needs to be seen straight away as anxieties are heightened. Families need to be seen, and treated with respect and honesty and not left in 'limbo'. There is no way of minimising this stressful time; however the best interests of the child are paramount for their health and safety.

Following baby Tony's strategy meeting, an initial assessment will be completed within seven working days and a recommendation made. This assessment is completed under the *Framework for the Assessment of Children and their Families* (Department of Health, 2000). If there is still concern then a child protection conference would be held to bring his parents and professionals together to share information, reports, discussion and plan how to safeguard this child following his non-accidental injury. Will the child be safe if he goes home? Sometimes parents or carers will agree that the child can be looked after by relatives whilst a risk assessment is completed over a period of 35 working days. If parents refuse then Social Care has the responsibility to seek legal advice to safeguard the child. This then actions orders from the court to assist the social care agency to continue to work with parents and carers within the legal framework.

In baby Tony's case the strategy meeting of professionals and the social worker's initial assessment highlighted the fact that Anna had not been present when this injury happened to her son, as she was at work. She had not delayed in presenting him at the hospital and agreed to work with professionals with a Core Assessment, over 35 working days. Her husband Robert was arrested and interviewed by the police and within that time he admitted that he had lost his temper with his baby son. He agreed to get help with his drink and temper problem. Anna decided that her son had to come first and that she would separate from her husband until he proved he had changed. A contract was signed by Anna that she would not leave their son on his own with his father and would continue to work within a family support plan with the social care staff. This contract is not legally binding. However if parents or carers do not work in partnership with the plan it can be a tool to take to court to show that they had a written explanation of why there was a need to work together, for the welfare of their child.

The enquiry into the death of Victoria Climbié, and the Chief Inspector's safeguarding reports brought forward the shortcomings of not intervening early enough, poor co-ordination, a failure to share information, and the absence of anyone with a strong sense of accountability. These informed the Green Paper entitled *Every Child Matters* and the Children Act 2004. The Department of Health published practice guidance to assist practitioners to work together to safeguard children from harm, known as 'What to do if you are worried a child is being abused' (DOH, 2006b).

Let's continue to communicate together and share our concerns so that all children are safeguarded.

The Radiographer's Perspective

Emily Hargreaves

Paediatric Team Leader

The role of the radiographer is to produce high-quality diagnostic images that contribute as evidence in the safeguarding of a child where abuse is suspected.

Due to high-profile cases and serious case reviews within social care, NAI skeletal survey examinations play an important part in investigations where abuse is suspected. The consultant paediatrician should discuss the referral with a consultant paediatric radiologist in order to justify the examination, giving clear details of the safeguarding concerns. The referral form should document the contact details of the referrer and social worker overseeing the child's care to aid communication before and after examination.

Local pathways should be in place to manage referral from the community (in cases where the child is deemed to be in a place of safety) or from the hospital ward (if the child has been admitted as a result of injury). Consent should be obtained by the referrer from the child's parent or legal guardian. Consent may be appointed by the court in cases where consent is withheld by the parent as the child is deemed vulnerable (Society and College of Radiographers, 2014). The radiographer should review the written consent before proceeding with the examination. A communication timeline can document as evidence any problems that cause a delay, from the time of referral to the examination.

The examination should routinely be performed within normal working hours by two suitably trained radiographers (Society and College of Radiographers, 2009). The radiographer should liaise with the nurse or social worker to ensure that they accompany the child. It is essential for them to be present, as they are responsible for the child's safety whilst in the department and they will act as a witness during the examination (Society and College of Radiographers, 2009). It is important for the parents to accompany the child, unless prohibited, as it is in the best interest of the child's welfare and wellness to have them present (Society and College of Radiographers, 2014). Parents can feel valued when assisting during the examination and can help distract the child.

Some parents can demonstrate anxiety and frustration through anger; others can be compliant and cooperate happily. It is essential to act professionally and not be judgemental, due to the nature of the examination. The radiographer must be calm, listen and recognise parents' feelings and respond appropriately. Introducing those involved and giving a thorough explanation of the examination can reassure parents and give them an opportunity to ask questions.

The examination should be performed in a designated room, prepared with immobilisation supports. The use of digital radiography equipment with correct paediatric exposure factors settings and image processing ensures that high-quality images are produced, while maintaining a low patient dose. Paediatric distraction aids should be available to assist in completing the examination. Music and sensory lights can have a calming effect on a child, and age-appropriate toys can distract and entertain them.

There is considerable variation in imaging protocols for skeletal surveys performed in the UK (Swinson et al. 2008). Local imaging protocols should be produced with the guidance of the British Society of Paediatric Radiology (see Table 1.1) and include image technique and criteria for each projection. It is inappropriate to perform a 'babygram' (one x-ray image including most of the baby), as the image will not be of the appropriate diagnostic quality. The so-called 'babygram' shows rotated limbs, poor definition of bony detail and reduced image sharpness (Offiah, 2008). It may not be necessary to repeat imaging of certain areas already performed within the last few days.

It is good practice to have one radiographer positioning the child for each projection, whilst the other manages the control panel and the image processing. The radiographers should take a systematic approach, maintaining the efficiency and speed of the examination in order to reduce distress to the child and parent to a minimum.

Table 1.1 **Imaging Guidelines**

Anatomy	Projection	Additional projections
Skull	AP and lateral.	Towne's view for occipital injury. SXRs should be taken with a skeletal survey even if a CT scan has been performed.
Chest	AP/frontal chest (including clavicles). Oblique views of the ribs (left and right).	
Abdomen	AP abdomen with pelvis and hips.	
Spine	Lateral spine – cervical and thoraco-lumbar.	
Limbs	AP humeri, AP forearms, AP femurs, AP tib/fib, PA hands and AP feet.	Lateral views of any suspected shaft fracture. Lateral coned views of the elbows/wrists/knees/ankles may demonstrate metaphyseal injuries in greater detail than AP views of the limbs alone. The consultant radiologist should decide this, when checking the films with the radiographers.

Clothing, wristbands and unused monitoring equipment should be removed to prevent image artefacts. The nappy should be removed when imaging the femur, abdomen and spine. Plaster cast applied causes artefact but can also restrict positioning for other projections. It is good practice to document reasons for any artefacts that are present, such as cannulas.

The 'As Low As Reasonably Possible' principle should be applied, showing evidence of collimation and lead gonad protection where applicable. The examination equates to 4 to 8 months of background radiation when adequate shielding is used (Royal College of Radiologists, 2008). Images should have physical markers present (Society and College of Radiographers, 2011).

Gentle immobilisation reduces movement unsharpness and improves image quality. Effective communication and providing clear information will encourage the parent to position the child's limbs by simple extension and holding, with no twisting movements

(Society and College of Radiographers, 2012). Sandbags can be used to immobilise the child's legs. Sponges can aid positioning to ensure that holders' fingers are not present in the images. Swaddling the child in a blanket can soothe them and limits the movement of the child's limbs for the skull x-rays. Take care when positioning a child with confirmed injuries – for instance, lay the child on the opposite side to a confirmed skull fracture.

Actively listen to the parents, explaining the progress of the examination and confirming their agreement to continue helping with the examination. A short break will allow the child to compose themselves if they are upset, and provides time to reflect before proceeding. Distraction techniques and constructive play should be used to reduce patient fear and anxiety, and sedation should be used in extreme cases (Society and College of Radiographers, 2012).

The radiographer is accountable for their actions during the examination. It is good practice to record projections, exposure factors, immobilisation aids and those present. Any safeguarding concerns or observations made during the examination should be documented and discussed with the appropriate staff. The child should not leave the department until a consultant radiologist has reviewed the images and is satisfied that a conclusive report can be made within 24 hours (Royal College of Radiologists, 2008).

A follow-up chest x-ray is required in 10–14 days to identify rib fractures that may not be visible at the initial examination. Other follow-up imaging may include projections of definite injuries or areas where injury is suspicious. Images may also be required of limbs out of plaster cast in order to date a fracture; this will involve liaising with the orthopaedics department.

The follow-up appointment should be at a convenient time for the parents to attend. It should be documented in the child's notes and in a letter to social care, and be included in the radiology report so it is communicated to all those involved in the child's care. Obtaining the social worker's details on the referral form allows the radiology department to liaise about follow-up appointments if the child's place of care has changed since discharge. A robust local procedure must be in place to notify the referring clinician if a child does not attend for the follow-up chest x-ray (Royal College of Radiologists, 2008).

For a radiographer, an NAI skeletal survey examination can be emotionally as well as technically challenging. It can be difficult to produce a significant number of images of high diagnostic quality on a paediatric patient, whilst effectively managing the parent's reactions and the child's emotions. For an optimal investigation, good communication with the multidisciplinary team responsible for the child's safeguarding is paramount.

Louise Lindsay spent six years working as a senior nurse in A & E and five years as an emergency nurse practitioner within the NHS. She is currently an ENP in a busy minor injury unit and is the unit's Link Nurse for child surveillance.

Joyce Clayton has been a social worker at St James University Hospital in Leeds for over 18 years, involved in child protection and child care social work. She has worked with the Child Development Team, Child Protection Team and is currently the Paediatric Hepatology Transplant Unit, Regional Paediatric Specialist Team Social Worker, a credited practice teacher, and works on call for the Emergency Duty Social Care Team.

Emily Hargreaves *qualified as a radiographer in 2008. Emily has recently been appointed team leader, overseeing the paediatric radiology department at Leeds Children's Hospital. She has a keen interest in improving the quality of images of paediatric patients, and works closely with the paediatric radiologist. She has audited the quality of neonates' chest x-rays, presented her findings within the Trust and instigated improved training in paediatric radiography. She is authorised to provide preliminary image interpretation of the appendicular skeleton for both adult and paediatric trauma patients. She has a special interest in child protection and non-accidental injury pathways.*

References

British Society of Paediatric Radiology (2015). http://www.mybspr.org/ (last accessed 8.11.2015).

Care Quality Commission (2015). http://www.cqc.org.uk (Accessed 8.11.2015). Search 'safeguarding protocol'.

Child Protection Health Advisory Group, Trustwide Child Protection Steering Group and the Leeds Named Nurses Child Protection Group (Sept 2002/2006). *Child Protection Policy/Child Protection Report Writing Guidelines*, Level 1 Child Protection E-Learning Module.

Cooper, M.A. (2000). 'Emergency Nurse Practitioners, Development of an Audit Tool' in *Emergency Nurse*, 8, (5): 34–9.

Department of Health (1999). *Working Together to Safeguard Children*, London: DH.

Department of Health (2000). *Framework for the Assessment of Children and their Families*, London: DH.

Department of Health (2006a). 'What to do if you're worried a child is being abused' in *Every Child Matters – Change for Children* (Non-Statutory Guidance), London: DH.

Department of Health (2006b). 'Working together to safeguard children, A guide to inter-agency working to safeguard and promote the welfare of children' in *Every Child Matters – Change for Children* (Statutory Guidance), London: Department of Health.

Dolan, K. (1997). 'Children in accident and emergency' in *Accident and Emergency Nursing*, 5 (2): 88–91.

Gay, J. (1992). 'A painful experience' in *Nursing Times*, 88 (25): 32–5.

Greenidge, P. (1997). 'Requesting and interpreting x-rays in A&E' in *Emergency Nurse*, 5 (5): 31–6.

Leeds Local Safeguarding Children Board (2007). Inter-Agency Child Protection Procedures. Managed by the Leeds Safeguarding Children Senior Co-ordinators on an ongoing basis, Leeds: LSCB.

Knipe, H. and Bhattacharya, B. *Non-accidental injuries.* http://radiopaedia.org/articles/non-accidental-injuries (accessed 3.10.2015).

Leeds Safeguarding Children Board (2007). West Yorkshire Safeguarding Procedures for Children, available at www.leedslscb.org.uk (last accessed 15.3.2008).

Leeds Teaching Hospital NHS Trust (2007). Paediatric Liaison Resource File. Produced by the Children Safeguarding Nursing Team within and managed by them on an ongoing basis, LTHT.

Leeds Teaching Hospital NHS Trust (2003). Policy for Referral of Patients to Radiology from Nurse Practitioners, Accident & Emergency/MIUs, LTHT.

Morgan, M. (1991). 'Nursing management of the injured child' reprinted in Davis, J. 'Children in accident and emergency, parental perceptions of the quality of care, Part 2' in *Accident and Emergency Nursing* (1995) 3 (2): 89–91.

National Society for the Prevention of Cruelty to Children (2004). *Child abuse in Britain*, available at www.nspcc.org.uk/html/home/whatwedo/childabuseinbritain.htm (last accessed 15.3.2008).

Offiah, A. (2008). An audit of skeletal surveys. *Clinical Radiology*. 63, 651–56.

Royal College of Paediatrics and Child Health (2010). *Safeguarding children and young people: roles competence for healthcare staff,* intercollegiate document.

Royal College of Radiologists (2008). Standards for Radiological Investigations of Suspected Non-accidental Injury. www.rcr.ac.uk/publication/standards-radiological-investigations-suspected-non-accidental-injury (last accessed 6.10.2015).

Society and College of Radiographers (2009). Skeletal Survey for Suspected NAI, SIDS and SUDI: Guidance for Radiographers. www.sor.org/learning/document-library/skeletal-survey-suspected-nai-sids-and-sudi-guidance-radiographers (last accessed 5.10.2015).

Society and College of Radiographers (2011). Imaging for non-accidental injury (NAI): use of anatomical markers. www.sor.org/learning/document-library/imaging-non-accidental-injury-nai-use-anatomical-markers (last accessed 6.10.2015).

Society and College of Radiographers (2012). Imaging Children; immobilisation, distraction techniques and use of sedation. www.sor.org/learning/document-library/imaging-children-immobilisation-distraction-techniques-and-use-sedation (last accessed 6.10.2015).

Society and College of Radiographers (2014). Guidance for Radiographers providing Forensic Services. www.sor.org/learning/document-library/guidance-radiographers-providing-forensic-radiography-services-0 (last accessed 5.10.2015).

Swinson, S., Tapp, M., Brindley, R., Chapman, S., Offiah, A. and Johnson, K. (2008). An audit of skeletal surveys for suspected non-accidental injury following publication of the British Society of Paediatric Radiology guidelines. *Clinical Radiology*. 63 (6): 651–56.

Tenenbein, M., Reed, M.H. and Black, G.B. (1990). The toddler's fracture revisited. *American Journal of Emergency Medicine*. 8, 208–11.

United Kingdom Central Council (1992a). *The Code of Professional Conduct for Midwives and Health Visitors.* London: UKCC.

United Kingdom Central Council (1992). *Scope of Professional Practice.* London: UKCC.

Whaley, L. and Wong, D. (1991). 'Nursing care of infants and children' reprinted in Wood, I. 'Communicating with children in A&E – what skills does the nurse need?' in *Accident and Emergency Nursing*, 1997, 5 (3): 137–41.

Wheeler, D. and Hobbs, C. (30 April 1988). Mistakes in diagnosing non accidental injury: 10 years' experience. Contemporary Themes. *British Medical Journal*. 296.

Wynne, J. (1994). 'The construction of child abuse in the accident and emergency department' in Clocke, C. *Health Visitors and Nurses*. Harlow: Longman, 75–87.

Youd, J. (2005). Lost generation. in *Emergency Nurse,* 12: 15–17.

2.

Introduction to paediatric fractures

Karen Sakthivel-Wainford

Children, infants and adolescents are not like 'little adults' with regard to trauma. Firstly, their bone structure and composition are different from those of adults. The skeleton of the young is more porous, less brittle, the Haversian canals are relatively large and their bones contain more water. This results in greater elasticity and plasticity of their bones, leading to various forms of incomplete fracture.

The periosteum in children also differs from that of adults. In a child the periosteum is thicker, more elastic and less firmly bound to bone. The fibres of Sharpey are less numerous and shorter in a child, resulting in them being less effective binders of the periosteum, leading to raised periosteum (in infection, NAI and trauma).

The thicker and more elastic periosteum is more likely to remain at least partially intact and attached to fracture fragments. Thus the periosteum in a child acts as a hinge between fracture fragments, assisting in the reduction and stabilisation of the fracture. Hence non-union in the child is quite rare.

Infants' bones consist of three types: elongated tubular bones, round bones (such as the carpal or tarsal bones) and sesamoid bones (in tendon and articular capsule). Elongated tubular bones are made up of three segments: paired metaphysis, paired epiphysis and diaphysis (shaft of the long bone).

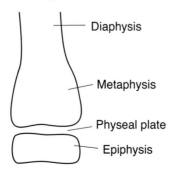

Figure 2.1 **Example of the end of a bone in an adolescent**

One of the most obvious differences between the skeleton of an adult and child is the degree of maturity. This can be seen by the presence of an epiphyseal ossification centre that is separated from the metaphysis of a long bone by a band of unossified cartilage (the physeal plate). The presence of these growth centres not only modifies the skeletal response to trauma but heightens concern because of the potential for growth disturbance.

The stress strain curve in children

Let us start by reviewing the stress strain curve for a paediatric bone. If a child falls with a certain amount of force, the bone will bend (due to the child's different bone structure, which gives the bone greater elasticity and plasticity). When the force is removed, the bone will return to its normal shape. This is called 'elastic deformation'. If the force with which the child falls is increased, there will come a 'yield point', at which the bone will bend but will not return to its normal shape. This is called 'plastic deformation' and results in a bow fracture. If the force of the trauma is further increased, the bone will reach a 'failure point', resulting in a complete fracture.

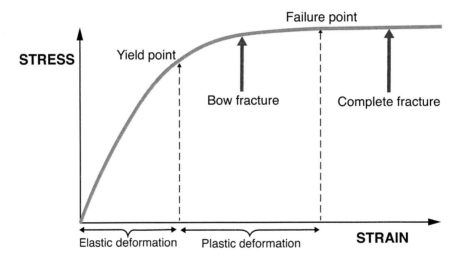

Figure 2.2 **Stress strain curve**

Incomplete fractures

Next, we shall look at some of the different types of incomplete fracture that children may experience following trauma.

Classic greenstick

The classic greenstick fracture is the result of a bending or angulation force that places the convex side of the bone in tension and the concave side in compression. This results in the tension forces producing an incomplete transverse fracture on the convex cortex, which extends to the middle of the shaft. The fracture involves half the bone, then turns at right angles at its most medial extent to create a vertical or longitudinal split. It is analogous to the fracture that would occur in a twig if bent.

Torus fracture

Torus is a Greek word meaning 'round swelling'. A torus fracture is a buckling of the cortex of the bone, produced by compression forces. It usually occurs in the metaphysis. A series of micro-fractures in the crystalline structure of young bones allow this buckling to occur. It is normally visualised on both the anterior posterior (AP) and lateral radiographs, although it may be more obvious on one image and extremely subtle on the other.

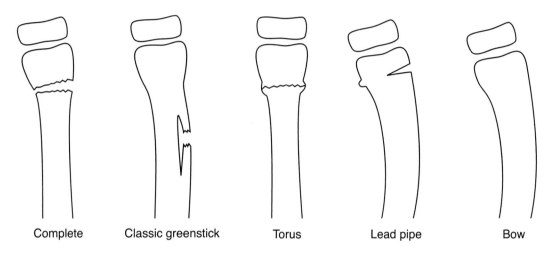

| Complete | Classic greenstick | Torus | Lead pipe | Bow |

Figure 2.3 **Incomplete and complete fractures in children**

Lead pipe

Lead pipe injury is analogous to the fracture that occurs in a lead pipe when bent. It occurs mainly in the metaphysis and is fairly uncommon. It combines an incomplete transverse fracture of one cortex and a torus fracture of the other side.

Bowing fracture

Due to the elasticity and plasticity of young bones, they may sometimes be bent without radiographic evidence of fracture. These are called bow fractures or plastic bowing fractures. They are a manifestation of plastic deformation as visualised on a stress strain curve (see Figure 2.2). The force involved exceeds the amount of elastic strain that would allow complete recovery of the normal shape, but is less than would be required to cause a complete fracture. They occur most commonly in the radius and ulna, but may also occur in the fibula (associated with a complete fracture of the tibia).

If the curvature is severe in the forearm, it may interfere with rotational movements. If the fibula is severely affected, it may interfere with proper alignment and apposition of an associated tibia fracture. Periosteal new bone formation is produced on the concave side, where histologically a series of micro-fractures occur. In younger patients (under 10 years of age), the bow fracture may be treated conservatively. Above this age, the orthopaediac surgeon may decide it is necessary to complete the fracture of the bone and surgically straighten it.

This leads us on to other types of fractures that occur in children and adolescents – injuries involving the physeal plate, and thus potentially causing growth disturbance. Firstly, we should clarify the difference between an apophysis and an epiphysis.

Apophyseal and epiphyseal injuries

The **epiphysis** is a secondary ossification centre situated adjacent to an articular surface and is responsible for the longitudinal growth of bones. Epiphyseal separation is analogous to dislocation or ligamentous injury in adults.

The **apophysis** is a secondary ossification centre *not* situated next to an articular surface and is responsible for growing bony projections or protruberances (usually for insertion of ligaments and tendons). Apophyseal separation is analogous to muscle pull or strain in adult.

As we have seen, the end of a bone is made up of an epiphysis, a physeal plate (also referred to as a physis, physeal line, epiphyseal plate, epiphyseal line and a metaphysis). All these terms originate from the Greek: *epi* meaning 'above', *meta* meaning 'adjacent' and *physis* meaning 'nature', from Homer's *Odyssey*, and they describe growth.

The physeal plate is made up of four distinct zones, starting from the metaphysis: zone one – resting or mother cells; zone two – proliferating cells; zone three – hypertrophic cells; zone four – provisional calcification. Zones one and two lie in the matrix and have collagen fibres running through, which strengthens these zones. Zone four (of provisional calcification) has some calcification and is therefore strengthened. However, zone three (the hypertrophic zone) is vulnerable to shearing forces so this is the area where physeal injuries occur. Fortunately, there is a separate blood supply to the epiphysis (from vessels within the joint) and the metaphysis (from vessels of the periosteum and nutrient vessel), so physeal injuries rarely cause avascular necrosis, apart from in the hip.

The joint capsule and ligamentous structures are 2–5 times stronger than the physeal plate. Hence trauma may result in fractures that involve the physeal plate, and these are normally classified according to the Salter Harris system (see Figure 2.4). This system of describing physeal injuries was first used in 1963 and is still widely used today. It is useful because it uses distinct radiographic patterns, each injury having clinical and prognostic significance.

The classification system divides fractures into five types, depending upon the pattern of involvement of the adjacent bone. All involve the physeal plate (see Figure 2.4). The classification system also indicates prognosis. The lower the number, the better the prognosis. (Hence Salter Harris type I and type II have a relatively good prognosis, whereas Salter Harris five fractures have a relatively poor prognosis.)

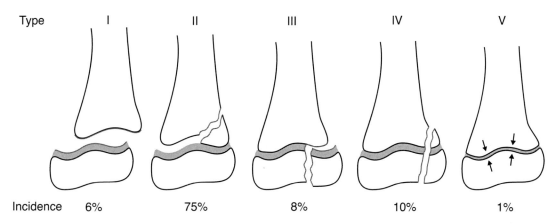

Figure 2.4 **Salter Harris classification and incidence**

As shown in Figure 2.4, Salter Harris I is a separation of the epiphysis and metaphysis at the physis, through the heterotrophic zone, and tends to occur in the younger child (below 10 years of age), when the physis is wider.

Salter Harris II is a separation at the physis and a fracture of the metaphysis, from a shearing and compression force. Salter Harris III is a fracture of the epiphysis, again involving physis, from a shear articular force.

Salter Harris IV is a fracture transversing the physis and involving the metaphysis and epiphysis, caused by a vertical split force, and can result in growth arrest and deformities. Salter Harris V is a compression of the physis, most common in 12–16 year olds. It may result in a shortened limb, as growth is arrested, due to the crushed physeal plate.

In total, 80 per cent of physeal plate injuries occur between 10 and 16 years of age, although Salter Harris type I fractures are more common in the under-ten age group. The joint capsule and ligamentous structures are stronger than the physeal plate. Hence in an adult a certain trauma may result in a ligamentous injury, whereas the same trauma in a child will often result in a physeal plate injury.

There are four other Salter Harris fractures, which are so rare that they are often not mentioned. Also it would be difficult, if not impossible, to assess them on plain radiographs. They are described below, for completeness:
- Type VI – an injury of the perchondral structure
- Type VII – an isolated injury to the epiphyseal plate

- Type VIII – an isolated injury to the metaphysis, with a potential injury related to endochondral ossification
- Type IX – an injury to the periosteum that may interfere with membraneous growth.

The cases in the following chapters will demonstrate many of these injuries, and may ask some questions about this chapter, so you can test yourself, to see if you have remembered the information, especially if it is all new to you.

3.

Overview of the limping child

Karen Sakthivel-Wainford

The presentation of a limping child, without clear history of trauma, to the A&E or MIU is a common occurrence. The child may be anywhere from 0 to 15 years of age; and the incidence is 2 in 1000 children per year. Limping in children often presents a clinical challenge.

Most cases are benign and self-limiting, such as transient synovitis. However, accurate assessment and treatment are essential, as other causes may be acute or life-threatening (such as septic arthritis) or chronic and disabling (such as Perthes disease).

Assessment may or may not involve x-ray images; other imaging modalities, such as ultrasound, may be more useful. This is where an agreed Trust pathway for the limping child is essential, to ensure the best outcome for the child.

Differential diagnosis

Firstly, what is the definition of a limping child? It is a deviation from the normal gait pattern, caused by pain, weakness or deformity. The patient often hurries off on one leg to offload a source of pain. Children do not have a reproducible gait until they are 7 years of age, so a subtle change in gait (or 'limp') may initially only be detected by close family.

The clinician will begin by categorising the limp according to age, acuity of presentation, etiology, type of gait disturbance and anatomical location. The clinician will also take a history, checking the patient's age, onset of symptoms, whether there is pain, and whether there has been a trauma or a systemic illness. Next they will examine the child, observe the child walking, take their temperature, and examine their lower legs, spine and abdomen.

From this, the clinician will start to rule to out some differentials, and make a list of possible differentials, which will then be a guide to the next step. The next step will probably be a decision as to whether or not imaging is required. If so, will it be x-ray or ultrasound?

At this stage, it will be helpful to look at a table to assess the primary differential diagnosis according to age.

Table 3.1 **Primary differential diagnosis of the limping child according to age**

0 to 3 years	3 to 10 years	10 to 15 years
Septic arthritis	Irritable hip	Slipped upper femoral epiphysis
Osteomyelitis	Septic arthritis	Septic arthritis
Development dysplasia of the hip	Osteomyelitis	Osteomyelitis
Fracture or soft tissue injury (stress fracture)	Perthes disease	Perthes disease
	Fracture or soft tissue injury (stress fracture)	Fracture or soft tissue injury (stress fracture)

A prospective study in Edinburgh reviewed 243 children presenting with a traumatic limp (Wynne-Davies and Gormley, 1978). The researchers found that hip pathology was the cause of the limp in over 60 per cent of the children; in 30 per cent there was no diagnosis. This highlights the fact that the most common cause of limping in children is pathology of the hip. The study found that the hip pathologies were due to irritable hip in 40 per cent of cases, unreported trauma in 16 per cent, Perthes disease in 2 per cent, and slipped upper femoral epiphysis in 1 per cent of cases.

As with any differential diagnosis, there are several other rare possible causes for a child's limp. These are listed below:
- Metabolic disease, such as rickets
- Differences in leg length
- Haematological disease, such as sickle cell
- Infections such as discitis or pyomyositis
- Neuroplastic disease, such as leukaemia
- Neuromuscular disease, such as cerebral palsy
- Rheumatological disease
- Intra-abdominal pathology and testicular torsion.

A brief overview of the most common causes of limping in children

This is just a brief look at the most common reasons for a child to limp. In the cases that follow this chapter there will be some examples of these, with more in-depth information provided in the answers to the cases – for example, clues to identifying slipped femoral epiphysis on an AP view.

Toddler's fracture

Toddler's fractures normally occur in preschool children, who are just learning to walk. The fall is often unwitnessed and involves a twisting action that results in an occult oblique fracture of the tibia, which is often seen on one x-ray image only. The fracture is sometimes not visualised on initial images. Follow-up images 10 days later may identify the fracture line as bone is reabsorbed along it. Signs of healing (i.e. callous formation) may also be seen.

On very rare occasions, other imaging modalities may be used to identify the fracture. However, one should consider the radiation dose to the child when discussing another imaging modality.

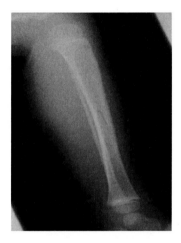

Figure 3.1 **Example of a Toddler's fracture only visible on lateral view**

Transient synositis

This is the most common cause of a traumatic limp and normally affects boys aged 4 to 8. It is a self-limiting disease and normally follows a viral infection. Diagnosis is based on a hip effusion demonstrated on ultrasound, and ruling out other causes. Hence there are no examples of this in the later cases.

Septic arthritis

This is an infection of the synovium and joint space. Factors that predict septic arthritis are a fever with a temperature over 38.5°C and an inability to weight bear. It often begins as a metaphyseal focus of osteomyelitis. Infections in children classically occur in the metaphysis, as the terminal blood vessels occur in loops with sluggish blood flow. In addition, there is a lack of phagocytes in the metaphyseal region.

When reviewing for osteomyelitis in a child radiographically, you are looking at the metaphysis for a lytic area, which may or may not have an accompanying periosteal reaction. The thin cortex of the metaphysis may be breached, allowing the infection to spread to the subperiosteal space, forming a periosteal abcess. If the metaphysis is intra-articular, involvement of the joint space may occur, resulting in septic arthritis.

Joint destruction and growth arrest may result from septic arthritis if it is left untreated. It is normally treated by urgent surgical washout and intravenous antibiotics.

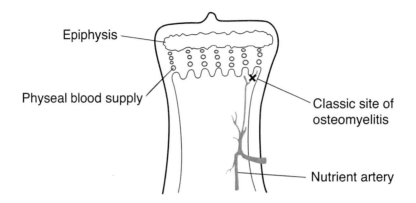

Figure 3.2 **Pathogenesis of long bone osteomyelitis**

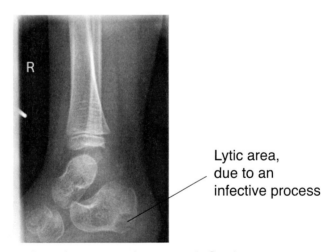

Figure 3.3 **Lytic area in calcaneum, due to an infective process**

Perthes disease

This normally occurs in boys aged 4 to 8, and is idiopathic avascular necrosis of the femoral head. Affected children are usually shorter than their peers and have a hyperactive tendency. The radiograph normally demonstrates sclerosis, flattening and fragmentation of the affected femoral epiphysis. A joint effusion may also be demonstrated. In the early stages it can be quite subtle, with minor sclerosis of the femoral epiphysis and associated joint effusion, often best visualised on the frog lateral view.

Treatment aims at containment of the hip within the acetabulum.

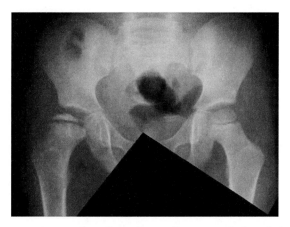

Figure 3.4 **Example of Perthes disease of the right hip**

Developmental dysplasia of the hip

Developmental dysplasia of the hip is the term that has replaced congenital dislocation of the hip. This is most common in girls. These days, it is usually diagnosed early, due to routine screening and selective ultrasound of high-risk groups. Plain radiographs of the hips will demonstrate this condition, and radiography is often carried out when there is late presentation.

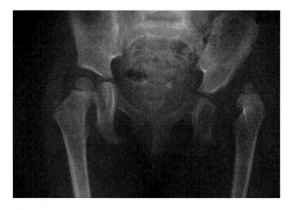

Figure 3.5 **Example of developmental dysplasia of the left hip**

Slipped upper femoral epiphysis (SUFE)

This usually affects children older than 10, and boys are more often affected than girls. The proximal femoral epiphysis displaces relative to the metaphysis; hence it is a Salter Harris type I injury.

33

Some of the risk factors are:
- Being overweight
- Being male
- Having endocrine anomalies, such as hypothyroidism or growth hormone deficiency
- Being Afro-Caribbean.

In 15 per cent of cases the patient can present with knee pain. The frog lateral view often confirms the diagnosis, following suspicions from the pelvis image.

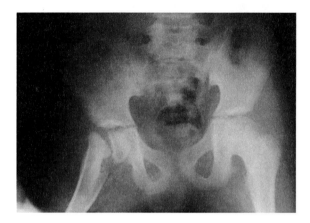

Figure 3.6 **Example of severe right hip SUFE, Salter Harris type injury**

The traumatic hip pathway

As previously mentioned, the most effective way to ensure correct diagnosis and management of this group of patients is for the medical teams to work together to produce a hip pathway, which is available for all.

Opposite is a copy of the Leeds NHS Trust pathway, which includes a list of 'red flags' for clinicians to watch out for.

Conclusion

It is vital to have a published limping child pathway in every NHS Trust. This pathway should be available for all to see, as a delay in diagnosis may worsen the outcome. Age is often a key factor when drawing up a list of differential diagnoses. The hip is the most common source of the pathology; however, there may be referred pain to the knee. All members of the multidisciplinary team should work together to reach the appropriate diagnosis, and high-quality appropriate imaging is often vital. The more knowledge we all have regarding how to review the x-ray image, the more likely it is that the correct diagnosis will be made.

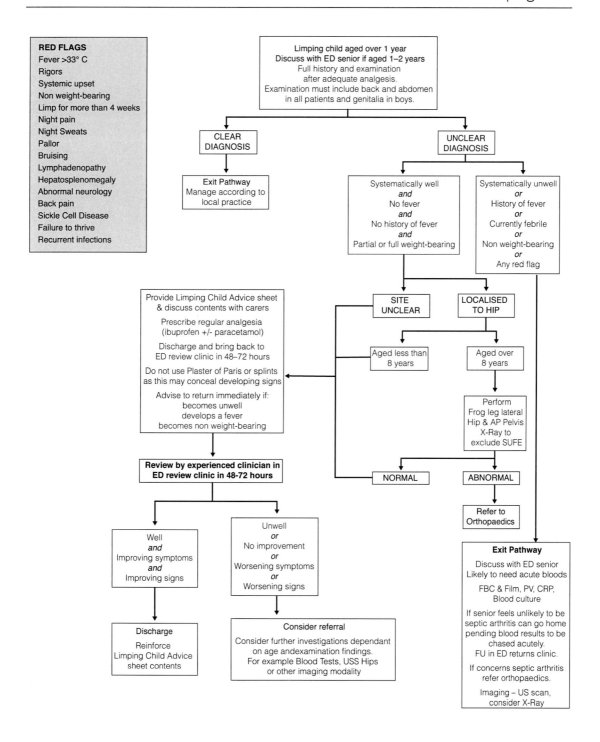

Figure 3.7 **The Leeds NHS Trust hip pathway for the limping child**

35

4.

Wrist and hand trauma

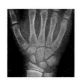

Case 1

Patient fell onto outstretched hand (FOOSH), now painful wrist.

Describe the radiographs.

In which of the three areas of long tubular bones is this type of injury normally located?

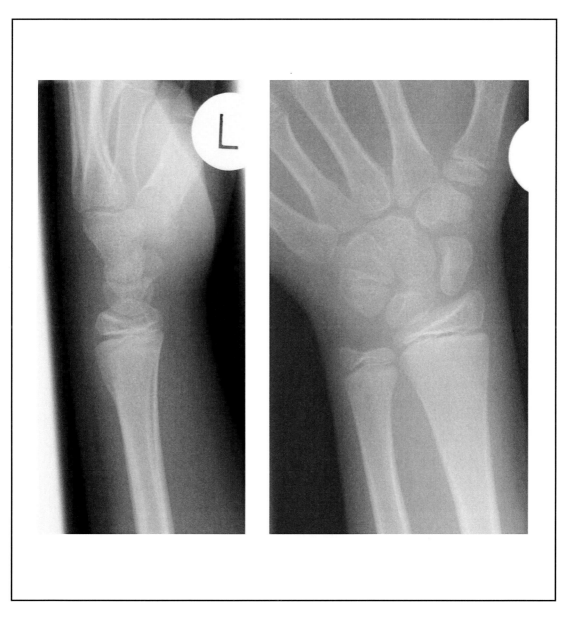

Answer to Case 1

There is a torus fracture of the dorsal aspect of the distal radial metaphysis. There is a loss in the normal volar angulation of the distal radius (normally volarly angulated by 10 to 15 degrees). Loss of the normal angulation of the distal radius is often a clue to injury. Torus fractures commonly occur in the metaphysis.

Torus is a Latin word meaning round swelling or protuberance. A torus fracture is a buckling of the cortex of the bone produced by compression forces. A series of micro-fractures in the crystalline structure of young bones allows this buckling to occur. When the child falls on their outstretched hand (as in this case) the buckling occurs on the dorsal aspect of the radius. If the child fell with the same amount of force causing the supinated hand to be compressed against the volar aspect of the wrist, then the torus fracture would be on the volar aspect of the wrist (a Smith's type fracture in an adult).

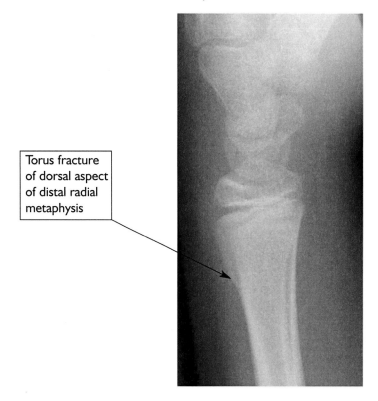

Torus fracture of dorsal aspect of distal radial metaphysis

Remember 'volar' refers to the anterior aspect of the forearm. It is essential when reviewing forearm radiographs that you look extremely carefully at the wrist and elbow as well as the length of the forearm, as many injuries occur at these joints.

In the young, the ends of the bones are often regarded as the weak areas due to the predominance of physeal plates there.

A fall on the outstretched hand results in different injuries depending on the age of the patient:

- under 5 years of age – supracondylar fracture of the distal humerus
- 5 to 10 years of age – transverse fracture of the metaphysis of the distal radius, 2 to 4 centimetres proximal to the growth plate (maybe an incomplete type fracture)
- 10 to 16 years of age – epiphyseal separation of the distal radius (most commonly a Salter Harris II)
- 18 to 35 years of age – fracture of the scaphoid or other carpal bone
- 40 years plus – a Colles type fracture.

These age ranges can be useful in the search for an injury, but remember they are meant only as guidelines, and children can have unusual or unexpected fractures for their age group.

Case 2

Patient fell from climbing frame, injuring wrist, unsure of mechanism of injury.

Describe the radiographs.

What is the name for this type of injury?

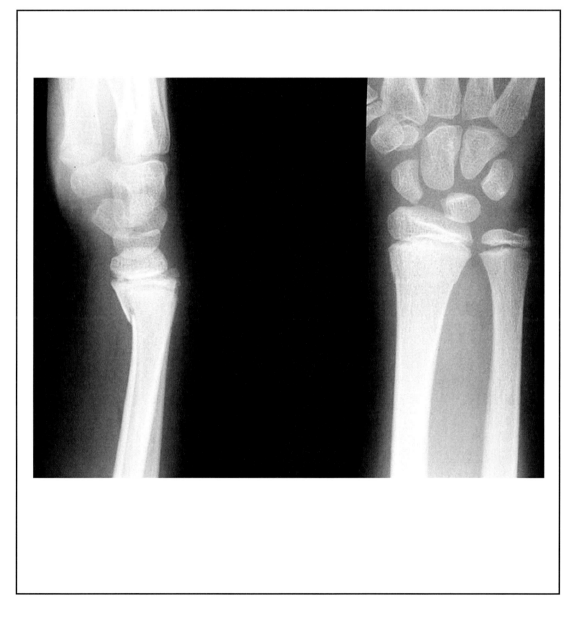

Answer to Case 2

There is a break in the cortex on the volar aspect of the distal radial metaphysis. This is a greenstick fracture. A classic greenstick fracture is a result of a bending or angulation force that places the convex side of the bone in tension and the concave side in compression.

This results in an incomplete transverse fracture being produced on the convex cortex by the tension forces which extends to the middle of the shaft, involving half the circumference of the bone, then turns at right angles at its most medial extent to create a vertical or longitudinal split. Often the longitudinal or vertical split is not visualised radiographically. This injury is meant to be like the bending of a twig, hence the name greenstick fracture.

Case 3

Patient fell onto outstretched hand, now painful wrist.

Describe the radiograph.

What is the name for this type of injury?

What is a bow type fracture, and where do they most commonly occur?

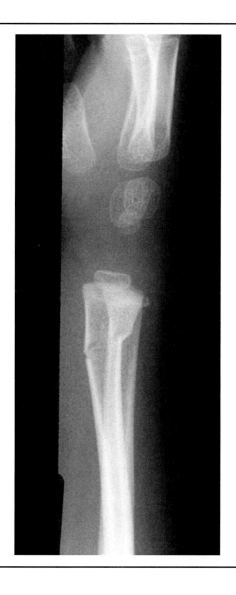

Answer to Case 3

Unfortunately there was no anterior posterior view available. There is an incomplete fracture of the volar aspect of the distal radius (metaphysis area), and a torus fracture of the dorsal aspect of the distal radius. This is called a 'lead pipe' fracture, analogous to the fracture that occurs in a lead pipe when bent. It is a fairly uncommon injury that normally occurs in the metaphysis and is a combination of an incomplete fracture of one cortex and a torus fracture of the other side. Note also there is dorsal angulation of the distal radius instead of the normal volar angulation.

Due to the normal elasticity and plasticity of young bones they may be bent without fracture; these are called bow fractures. If a child's bone is bent with a certain amount of force it will bend and return to normal; this is called elastic deformation. If you increase the force then the bone will bend and stay bent; this is plastic deformation and results in a bow fracture. Some authors represent this phenomenon by a stress/strain curve. If you increase the force further on the bone then you reach failure point and this results in a fracture. To conclude, with a bow fracture the force involved exceeds the amount of elastic strain that allows complete recovery of the normal shape but is less than is required to cause a complete fracture. Bow fractures occur most commonly in the radius and ulna, but may also occur in the fibula. If the curvature is severe in the forearm it may interfere with rotational movements. If the fibula is severely affected it may interfere with proper alignment and apposition of an associated fracture of the tibia. Periosteal new bone formation is produced on the concave side, where histiologically a series of microfractures occur.

Case 4

Patient was playing netball, and hyperextended the thumb.
Now pain in thumb.

Describe the radiographs.

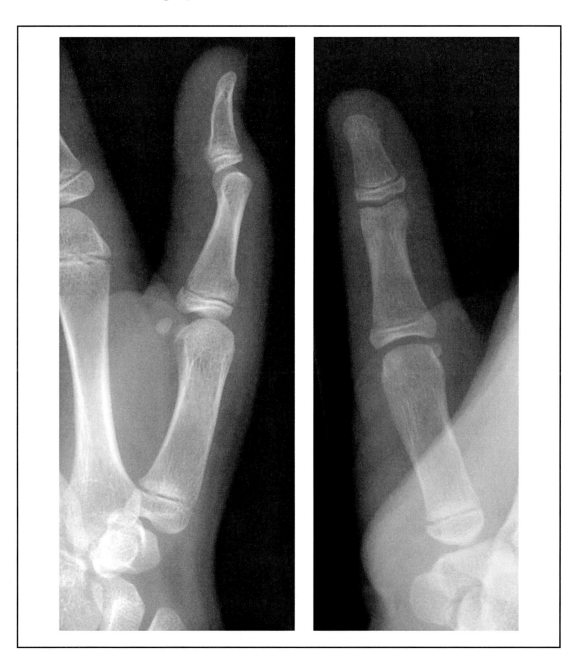

Answer to Case 4

There appears to be a torus type fracture (a buckling of the metaphysis) on the dorsal aspect of the proximal phalanx metaphysis. However on closer inspection at the site of the torus fracture there is a lucent line that probably transverses into the physeal plate. A fracture that involves the physeal plate and the metaphysis is classified as a Salter Harris II fracture (see Case 5 for Salter Harris classification).

The physeal plate is made of four distinct zones, starting from the metaphysis: zone 1 is resting/mother cells, 2 is proliferating cells, 3 is hypertrophic cells, 4 is area of provisional calcification. Zones 1 and 2 lie in the matrix and have collagen fibres running through, which strengthens these zones. Zone 4 has some calcification hence is strengthened. The hypertrophic zone, however, is vulnerable to shearing forces, hence this is the area where physeal injuries occur. Fortunately there is a separate blood supply to the epiphysis (from vessels within the joint) and the metaphysis (from vessels of the periosteum and nutrient vessel), so physeal injuries rarely cause avascular necrosis apart from in the hip (see hip cases in Chapter 9).

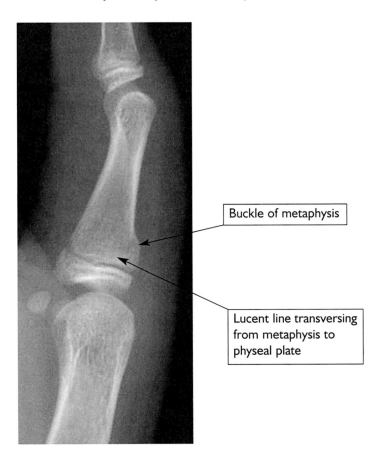

Buckle of metaphysis

Lucent line transversing from metaphysis to physeal plate

Case 5

Patient injured thumb in a rugby tackle, now painful thumb.

Describe the injury using Salter Harris classification.

Describe the five Salter Harris classifications, commenting on which areas of the bone they involve (for example, the metaphysis, and/or epiphysis).

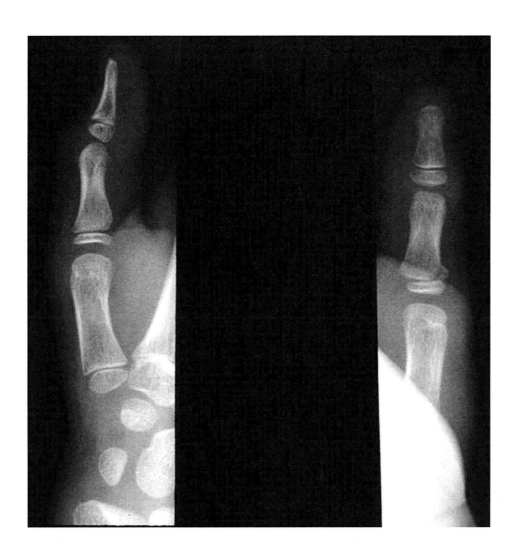

Answer to Case 5

There is a fracture transversing the metaphysis of the proximal phalanx into the physeal plate, radial aspect; this was classified by Salter and Harris as a Salter Harris II.

Salter and Harris first described physeal injuries in 1963. Their classification system is extremely useful as it uses distinct radiographic patterns, and each injury has a clinical and prognostic significance. There are in fact up to nine types of Salter Harris fracture, but the most common are the five basic types shown below.

The classification system divides fractures into five types, depending upon the pattern of involvement of the adjacent bone; all involve the physeal plate (see Figure 2.4, p. 27). The classification system also indicates prognosis – the lower the number the better the prognosis (hence Salter Harris I and II have a relatively good prognosis, whereas Salter Harris V fractures have a relatively poor prognosis).

As demonstrated in Figure 2.4 (p. 27), type I is a separation of the epiphysis and metaphysis at the physeal plate, type II is a separation at the physeal plate and a fracture of the metaphysis, type III is a fracture of the epiphysis, again involving physeal plate, type IV is a fracture transversing the physeal plate and involving the metaphysis and epiphysis, and type V is a compression of the physeal plate.

Eighty per cent of physeal plate injuries occur between the ages of 10 and 16 years of age, although Salter Harris I fractures are more common in the under 5s. The joint capsule and ligamentous structures are stronger than the physeal plate. Hence in an adult a certain trauma may result in ligamentous injury whereas the same trauma in a child will often result in a physeal plate injury.

The other four types of Salter Harris fractures are rare and often not mentioned, but for completeness are described.

- type VI – consists of an injury to the perichondral structures
- type VII – is an isolated injury to the epiphyseal plate
- type VIII – is an isolated injury to the metaphysis, with a potential injury related to endochondral ossification
- type IX – is an injury to the periosteum that may interfere with membranous growth.

Case 6

Patient banged thumb on a piece of furniture, now painful and swollen.

Describe the radiographs.

What lies directly above the physeal plate of the distal phalanx of the hands and feet? What is the importance of this?

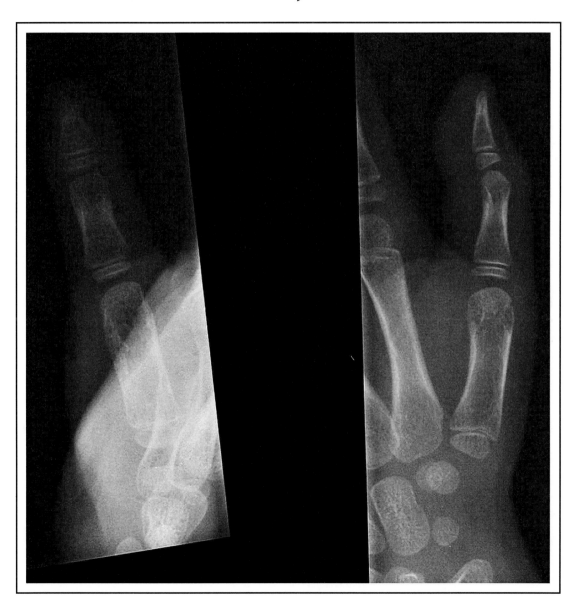

Answer to Case 6

There is a widening of the physeal plate of the distal phalanx dorsally (demonstrated on the lateral radiograph). If you look closely there is a small flake of bone at the physeal plate which has come from the metaphysis, hence this is a Salter Harris type II injury. More commonly the mechanism of injury in this case results in a Salter Harris I of the distal phalanx.

Above the physeal plate of the distal phalanx is the nail bed, hence it may be an open injury resulting in osteomyelitis if no antibiotic cover is given.

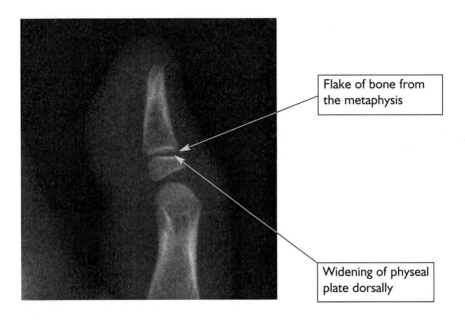

Flake of bone from the metaphysis

Widening of physeal plate dorsally

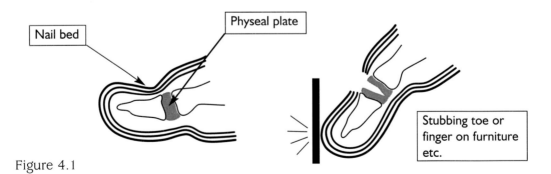

Nail bed

Physeal plate

Stubbing toe or finger on furniture etc.

Figure 4.1
Occult, open Salter Harris type I injury

Case 7

Patient fell injuring hand, bony tenderness mainly to little finger.

Describe the radiographs.

Is there an injury? If so, classify.

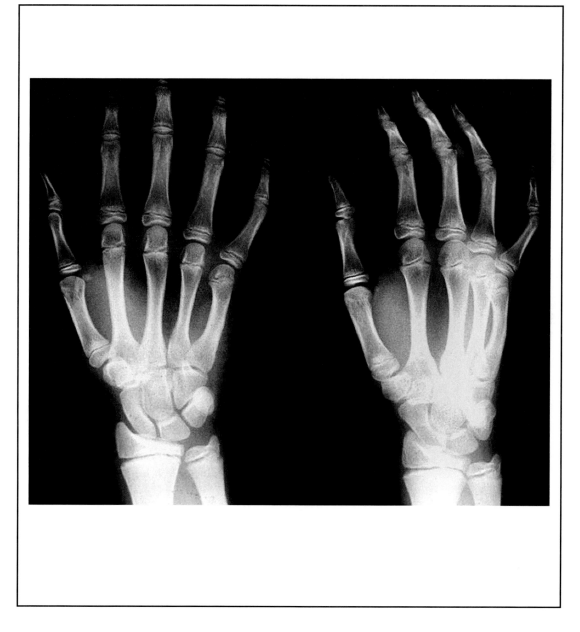

Answer to Case 7

There is a break in the cortex and a lucent line at the metaphysis of the proximal phalanx, little finger ulnar aspect. The lucency travels from the metaphysis to the physeal plate; this is a Salter Harris II fracture. Physeal injuries are relatively common at the heads of metacarpals and bases of the proximal phalanges of the hands. This is an area of numerous physeal plates making it potentially a weak area in the hands. This type of injury is often difficult to visualise, requiring magnification and sometimes windowing on the PACS monitor. They are best demonstrated on the oblique radiograph. In children, the proximal phalanx is involved in over 50 per cent of fractures of the phalanx.

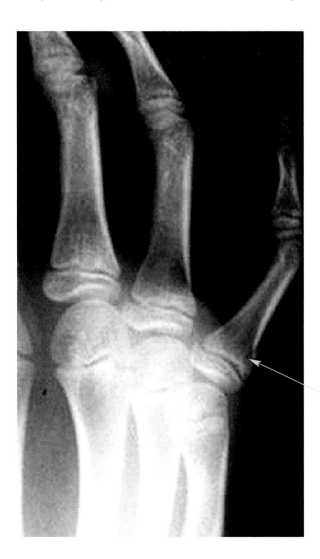

Lucent line transversing metaphysis entering physeal plate = Salter Harris II; also small buckle of cortex here

Case 8

Patient fell on outstretched hand.

Describe the injury.

Should another view be considered?

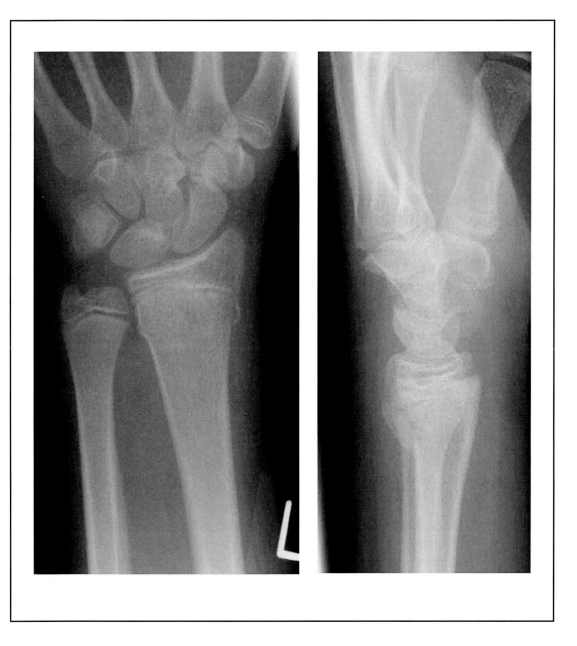

Answer to Case 8

The posterior anterior view demonstrates a buckling of the cortex of the distal radius at the metaphysis. The lateral view clearly demonstrates a break in the cortex of the distal radius at the metaphysis; there is also slight dorsal angulation of the distal radius (instead of the normal volar angulation). On reviewing the lateral radiograph the fracture line probably enters the physeal plate, hence it is a Salter Harris II fracture (although difficult to visualise on this radiograph). Also there is widening of the volar aspect of the physeal plate (hence the physeal plate is involved). On a normal lateral radiograph the radius overlies the ulna which can sometimes make it difficult to view the dorsal metaphysis of the distal radius (as in this case). A radiograph with the hand slightly supinated will clear the dorsal radial border away from the ulna, demonstrating this area more clearly. Whether another view with the hand slightly supinated is carried out depends on whether it will alter patient management, local protocols, and the additional radiation dose to a young child.

When there is high suspicion of a fracture in this area, which is not demonstrated sufficiently on posterior anterior and lateral views, this additional oblique view should be considered in order to prevent missing a fracture.

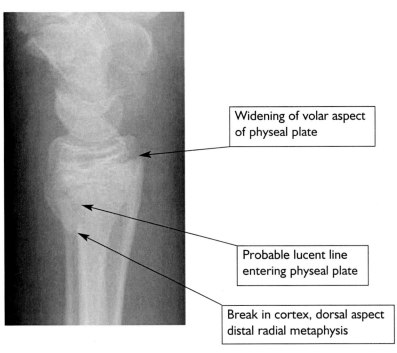

Widening of volar aspect of physeal plate

Probable lucent line entering physeal plate

Break in cortex, dorsal aspect distal radial metaphysis

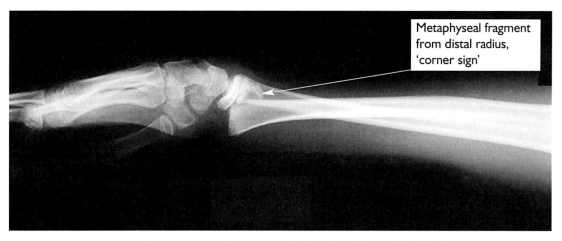

Figure 4.2 **Salter Harris II fracture of distal radius with displacement**

The most common site of epiphyseal injury is the distal radius, resulting from a fall on an outstretched hand. It may not be readily viewed on the posterior anterior radiograph. However on the lateral radiograph a fracture of the dorsal, distal radial metaphysis with widening of the volar physeal plate may be visualised (the 'corner sign'). Care is required in assessing this injury as the metaphyseal fragment may be undisplaced, due to the relative strength of the surrounding ligaments returning the metaphyseal fragment to its normal place when the force is removed. If the patient falls supinating their hand against their wrist then the metaphyseal fragment will be on the volar aspect of the radius, with widening of the dorsal aspect of the physeal plate (a Smith's type fracture in an adult).

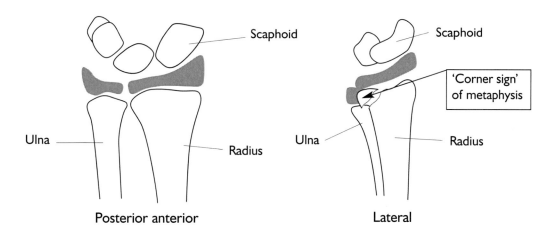

Figure 4.3 **Salter Harris II fracture of the distal radius from a fall on outstretched hand**

Case 9

Patient hit a wall with fist, now pain in fifth metacarpal (little finger metacarpal).

Describe the radiographs.

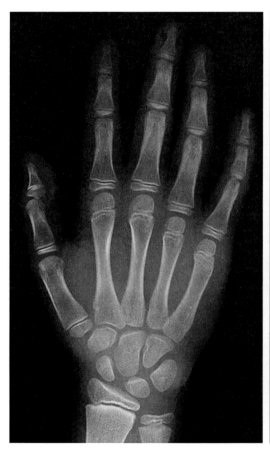
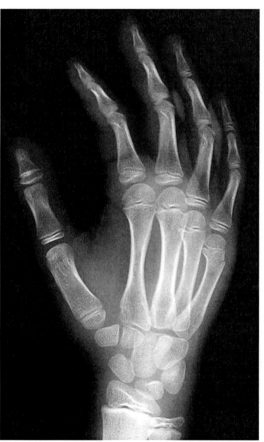

Answer to Case 9

The posterior anterior view demonstrates a small buckle in the cortex of the fifth metacarpal (little finger) at the metaphysis. Often paediatric fractures are subtle, and it is useful to review many normal radiographs of each area so that it is easier to notice subtle buckles when they occur. In this case the oblique radiograph readily demonstrates the fracture. There is a break in the cortex of the dorsal aspect of the metaphysis of the fifth metacarpal (little finger); this is a greenstick fracture. New thinking suggests that instead of the fifth metacarpal we call it the little finger metacarpal, etc., to avoid confusion.

This buckle fracture in children would, in an adult, become a fracture of the neck of the fifth metacarpal (little finger metacarpal), commonly known as the 'boxer's fracture'.

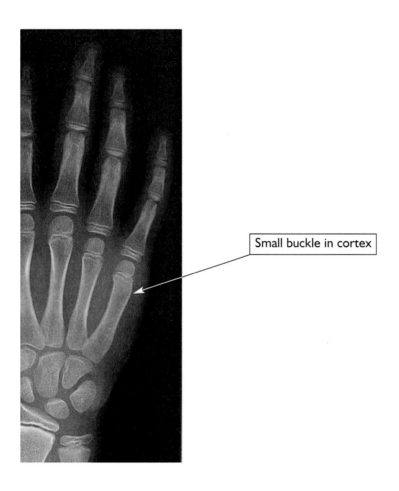

Small buckle in cortex

Case 10

Patient fell in games at school, painful deformed finger.

Describe the radiographs, and classify.

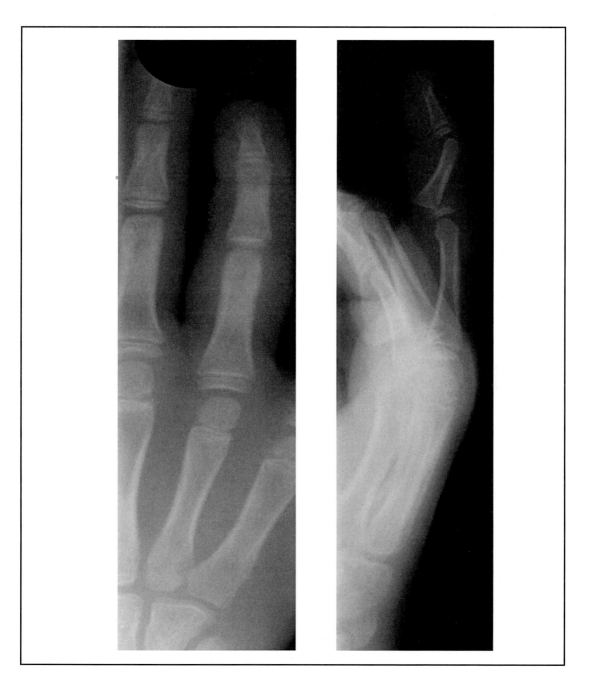

Answer to Case 10

The posterior anterior view does not demonstrate the injury, which highlights the necessity of always reviewing two radiographic projections of the affected area at right angles to each other. The lateral view readily demonstrates the gross separation at the physeal plate, of the middle phalanx with volar displacement of the metaphysis. Two fragments of bone are present at the physeal area, one at the volar aspect, the other dorsal. These fragments of bone are probably from the metaphysis, hence this is a Salter Harris type II injury.

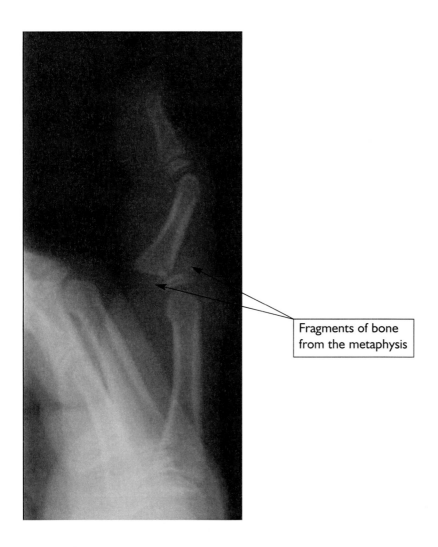

Fragments of bone
from the metaphysis

Case 11

Patient hyperextended finger in netball. Now painful finger and appears deformed.

Describe the radiographs.

Is there an injury?

Describe a common injury to the finger from hyperextension.

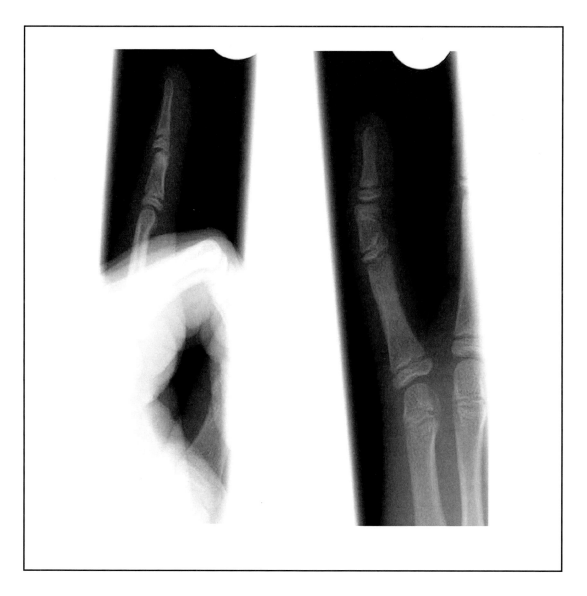

Answer to Case 11

The patient has a shortened middle phalanx with what appears to be an angulated, accessory physeal plate distally, which results in the finger being angulated. This is clinodactyly of the fifth finger (Keats has a similar example in his book of normal variants). The clinician, on discussion with the child and mother, came to the conclusion that the finger was no more angulated than normal, plus the fifth finger on the other hand was the same. Be careful when reviewing paediatric hand radiographs as they can have accessory ossification centres and false ossification centres (particularly at the base of the metacarpals).

No injury was seen on the radiographs. A common injury from hyperextension of the finger is an avulsion of the volar aspect of the middle phalanx, a volar plate type avulsion.

Clinodactyly is a shortened middle phalanx (which may be angulated as in this case), whereas Kirner's anomaly is a shortened distal phalanx.

Case 12

Patient fell on outstretched hand, now painful wrist.

Describe the radiographs.

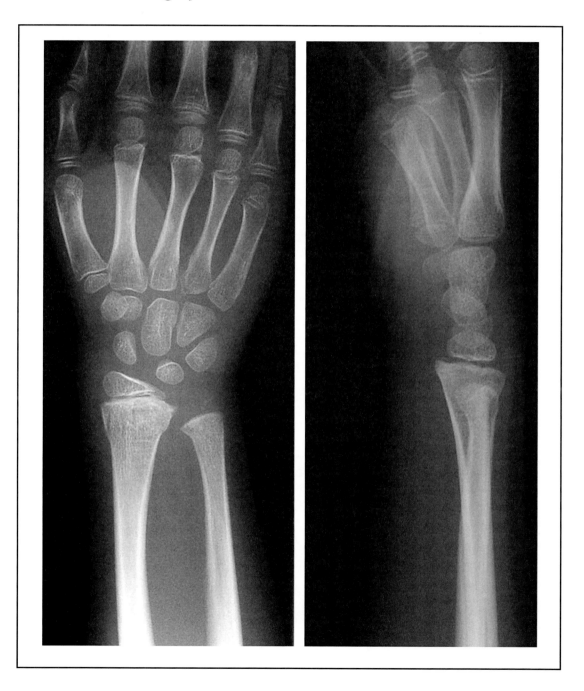

Answer to Case 12

On the anterior posterior radiograph a small buckle of the distal radius is visible. Also demonstrated is a buckle (torus) type fracture of the distal ulna. The lateral view demonstrates the torus fracture of the distal radius on the dorsal aspect; there is also dorsal angulation of the distal radius. Remember the distal radius is normally angulated volarly (10 to 15 degrees), and ulnarly (17 degrees) – alteration in this is a clue to injury. The torus fracture of the distal ulna is also demonstrated on the lateral view (remember to look through the radius to the ulnar on the lateral).

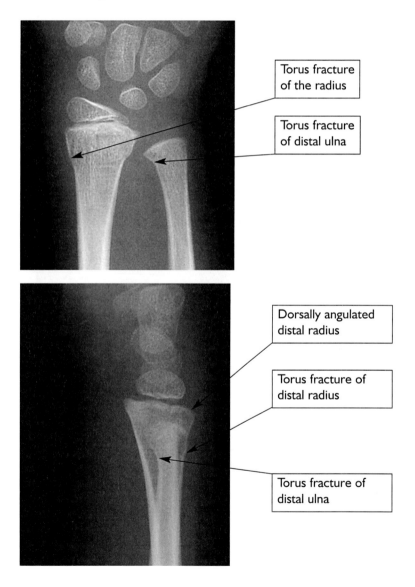

Torus fracture of the radius

Torus fracture of distal ulna

Dorsally angulated distal radius

Torus fracture of distal radius

Torus fracture of distal ulna

Case 13

Patient fell from bike, injuring hand.

Describe and classify the injury.

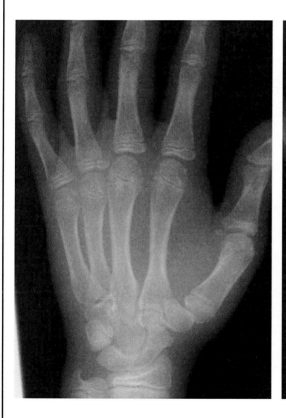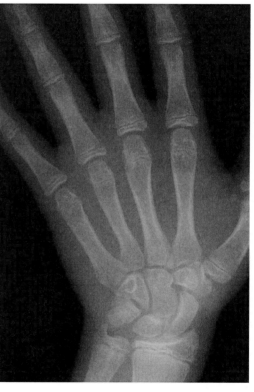

Answer to Case 13

There is a vertical lucent line through the epiphysis of the proximal phalanx of the ring finger, with widening of the physeal plate, radial aspect. This is a Salter Harris type III injury. However on closer inspection of the oblique view (this type of injury is frequently more clearly demonstrated on the oblique view), a small fragment of the metaphysis, radial aspect of proximal phalanx is noted, hence this would make it a Salter Harris type IV injury.

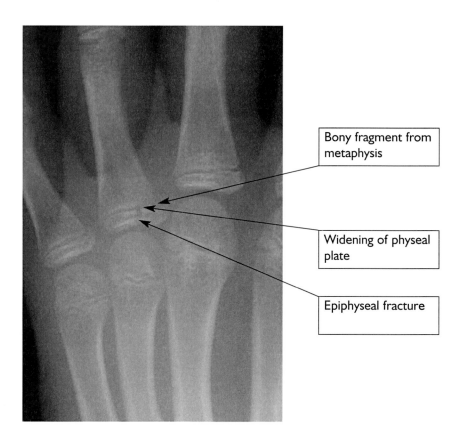

Bony fragment from metaphysis

Widening of physeal plate

Epiphyseal fracture

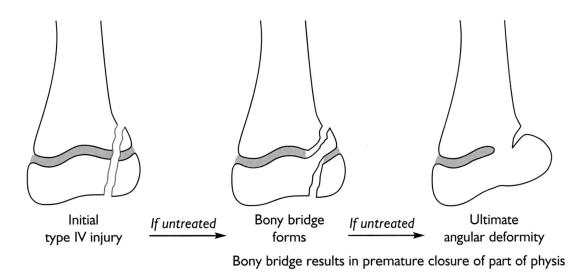

Figure 4.4 **Growth disturbance in Salter Harris type IV injuries**

A problem with Salter Harris type IV injuries is that callus formation may occur across the physeal plate leading to premature closure of part of the physeal plate, resulting in an angular deformity of that bone at the joint. It is therefore imperative that Salter Harris type IV injuries are radiographically visualised and accurately reported to ensure correct management. Salter Harris type IV injuries are normally caused by a vertical splitting force. Even with careful management growth arrest and joint deformities are possible.

Case 14

Patient hyperextended finger whilst playing netball.

Describe the radiographs.

If an adult had the same mechanism of injury, what type of injury would you be looking for?

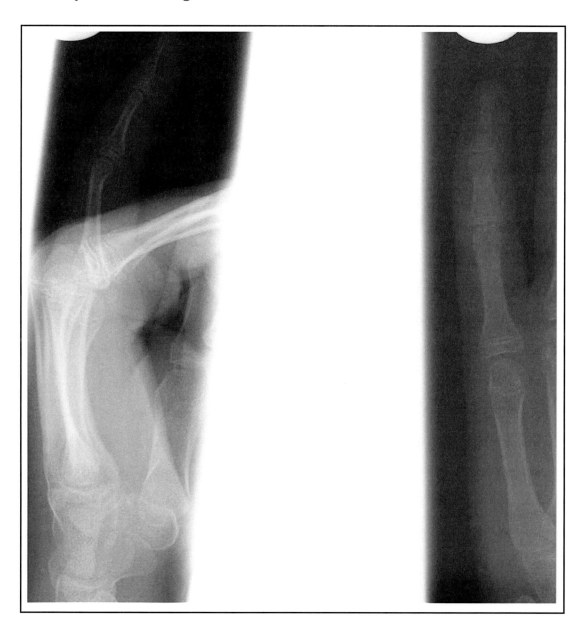

Answer to Case 14

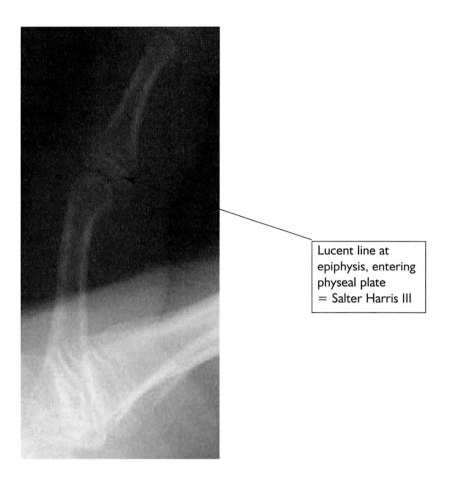

Lucent line at
epiphysis, entering
physeal plate
= Salter Harris III

There is a lucent line volar aspect of epiphysis of middle phalanx entering into the physeal plate, hence it is Salter Harris type III injury, involving about a third of the articular surface. Injuries involving more than a third of the articular surface often need more careful management to prevent early arthritis.

If an adult hyperextended their finger the most likely injury would be an avulsion of the volar aspect of the middle phalanx at the proximal interphalangeal joint (volar plate avulsion). This is due to the fact that in adolescence the physeal plate is much weaker than the ligaments or bone, hence with the same mechanism of injury an adult will receive a ligament or bony injury, whereas an adolescent will have a physeal injury (often involving nearby bone as well – as in this case).

Case 15

Patient fell during games at school palmar flexing hand, now pain in wrist.

Describe the radiographs.

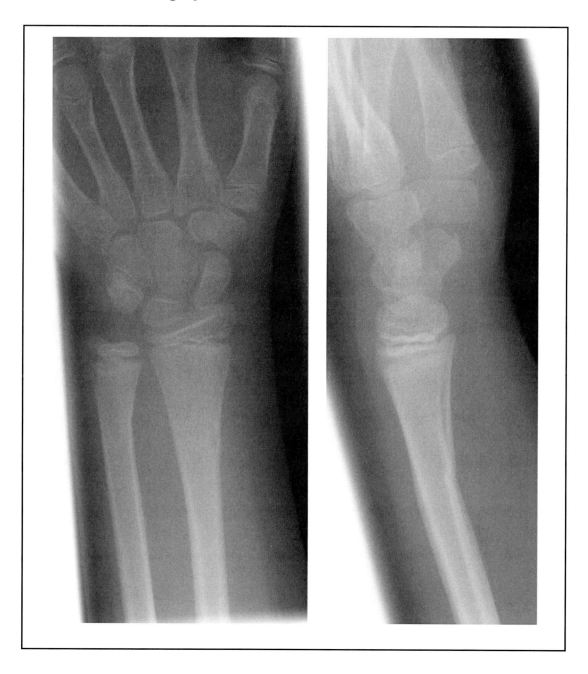

Answer to Case 15

There is torus type fracture of the distal radius, demonstrated on the lateral view on the volar aspect, due to compression of the trabeculae (if this had been an adult it would have resulted in a Smith's type fracture). If the patient had fallen on their outstretched hand the torus fracture would have been on the dorsal aspect of the distal radius (in an adult this would have resulted in a Colles fracture).

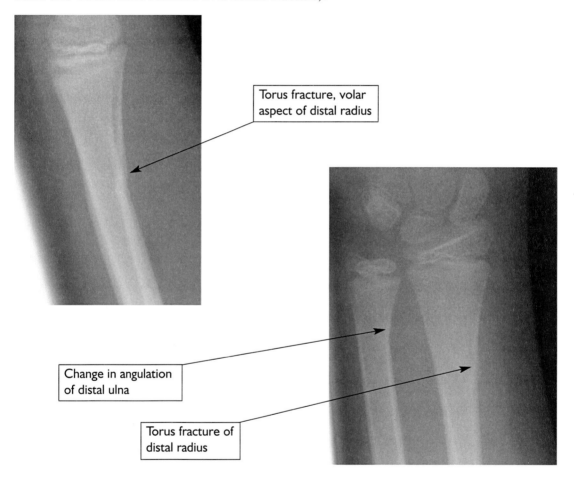

Torus fracture, volar aspect of distal radius

Change in angulation of distal ulna

Torus fracture of distal radius

The posterior anterior view demonstrates the torus fracture of the distal radius, but also demonstrates a sharp angulation of the distal ulna cortex, lateral aspect instead of the normal smooth curvature, slightly more distal than the radial fracture. This is a buckle type fracture of the distal ulna. Torus/buckle fractures are often very subtle, hence it is useful to review many normal paediatric radiographs in order to better appreciate subtle changes in alignment (see Case 75).

Case 16

Patient fell onto outstretched hand, now painful carpus and distal radius. However, there is no bony tenderness to the scaphoid.

Provide a provisional evaluation of the images.

Is there a fracture?

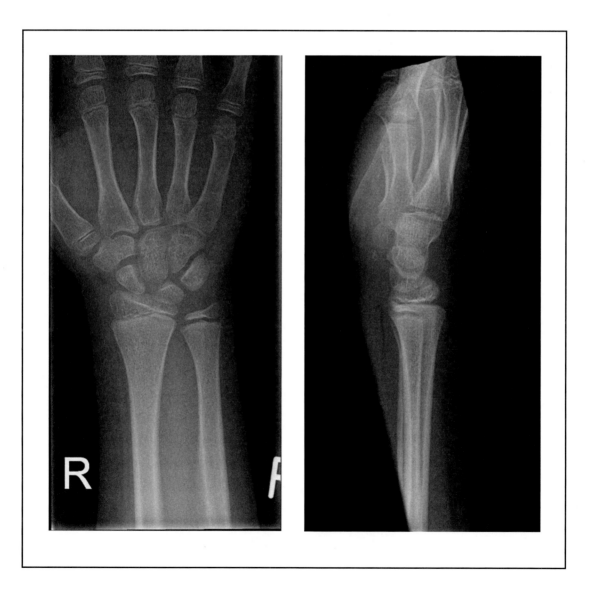

Answer to Case 16

There is no bony injury demonstrated. However, a fragmented pisiform at the volar aspect of the carpus is visualised. This is normal; the pisiform is often fragmented early in its development and can be mistaken for a fracture. If the lateral radiograph is slightly supinated (as in this case), the pisiform is easier to visualise and appears more volar placed than normal, but this is just projectional.

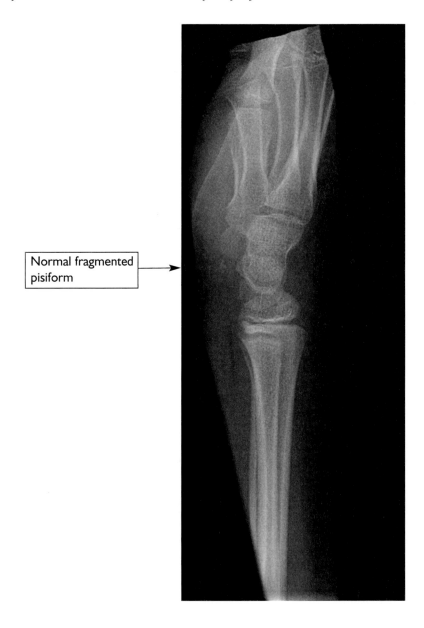

Normal fragmented pisiform

Case 17

Adolescent hit a wall, now bony tender proximal phalanx.

Write a provisional image evaluation.

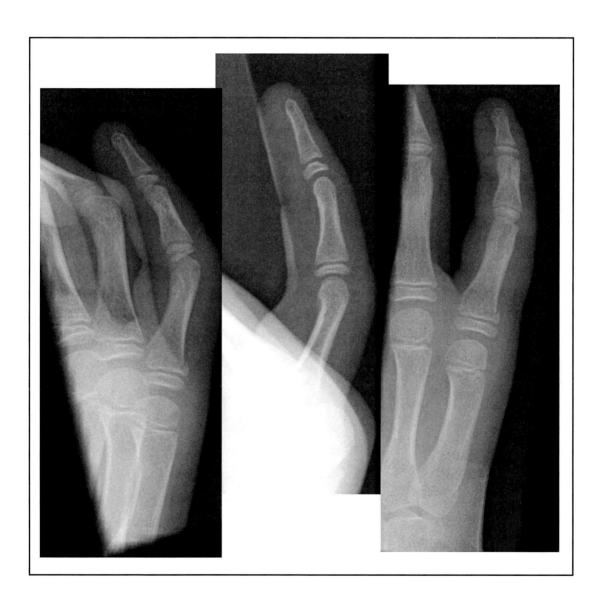

Answer to Case 17

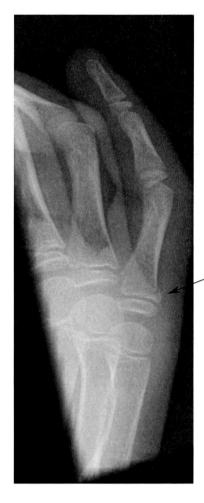

Salter Harris II fracture; also transverse fracture of the base of proximal phalanx

The DP demonstrates a Salter Harris type II fracture of the ulnar aspect of the base of the proximal phalanx of the little finger. However, on reviewing the oblique view (as seen above), there is also a transverse fracture of the metaphysis of the base of the proximal phalanx, with radial/volar displacement of the distal part. Remember, you always describe what is happening to the distal part of the bone. This example highlights how useful oblique views are, especially when reviewing the proximal phalanx in children. In the departments where I work, if the paediatric patient is bony tender at the proximal phalanx, and the requesting clinician suspects a fracture of the proximal phalanx, then we routinely do an oblique view of the area. In this case, the fracture could be identified on the DP view, but not its full extent. Often the fracture is difficult to identify on the DP, but is easily visualised on the oblique view.

Case 18

Patient fell on outstretched hand, bony tender distal radius.

Write a provisional image evaluation.

Would another projection be helpful?

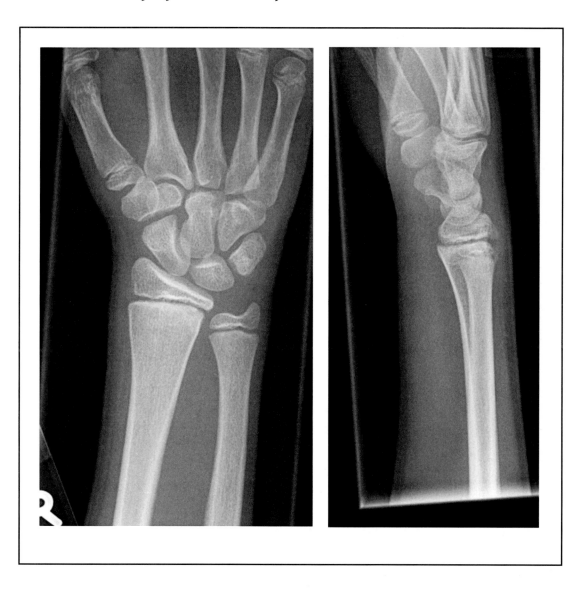

Answer to Case 18

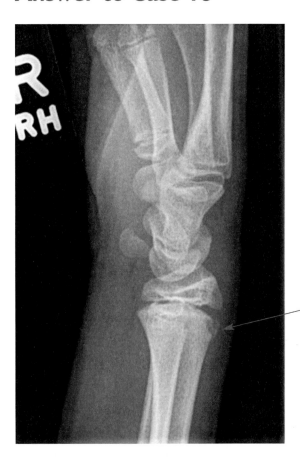

Salter Harris type II fracture at dorsal aspect of distal radius, more easily identified on slightly supinated wrist view

The lateral view of the wrist raises the suspicion of a Salter Harris type II fracture of the distal radius, the so-called 'corner sign', which would fit with the clinical details. On seeing this appearance, the radiographer did a slightly supinated wrist view, which moves the ulnar volarly away from the dorsal aspect of the distal radius, allowing better visualisation of the dorsal aspect of the distal radial metaphysis. This additional view confirmed a definite Salter Harris type II fracture of the distal radius. This is a useful projection to remember when reviewing wrist images for subtle Salter Harris type II fractures.

Case 19

Fell onto outstretched hand, bony tender distal radius.

Write a provisional image evaluation.

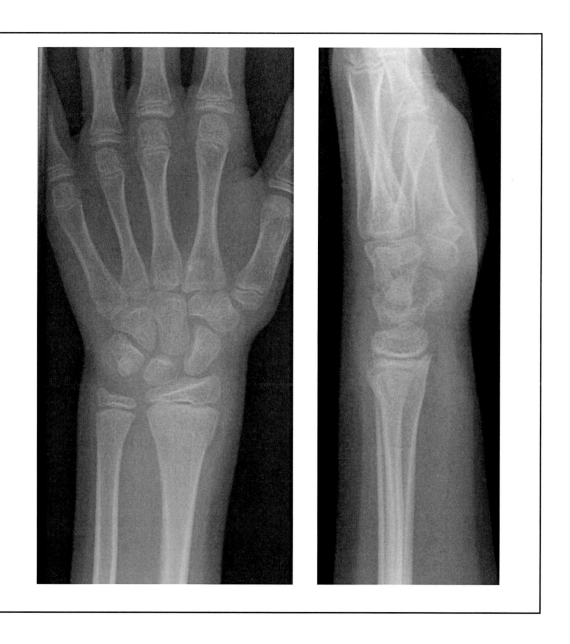

Answer to Case 19

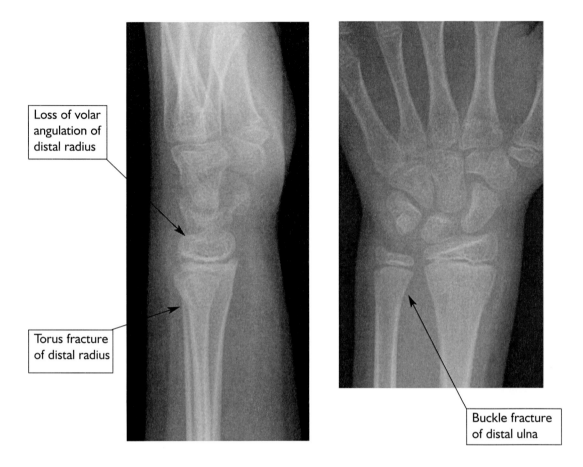

Loss of volar angulation of distal radius

Torus fracture of distal radius

Buckle fracture of distal ulna

There is a torus fracture of the distal radial metaphysis, with some dorsal angulation of the distal part, plus associated buckle fracture of the ulnar metaphysis. Torus fractures are normally demonstrated on both x-ray images, resembling the bulbous tops of Greek columns. However, buckle fractures are more subtle, only demonstrated on one x-ray image, and represented by an angular appearance to the smooth curve of a long bone. Buckle fractures may be seen accompanying incomplete fractures of the distal radius, if the images are carefully reviewed.

Case 20

Hyperextension of little finger in netball. Bony tender all of little finger.

Write a provisional image evaluation.

Which areas are most likely to be injured in a hyperextension injury?

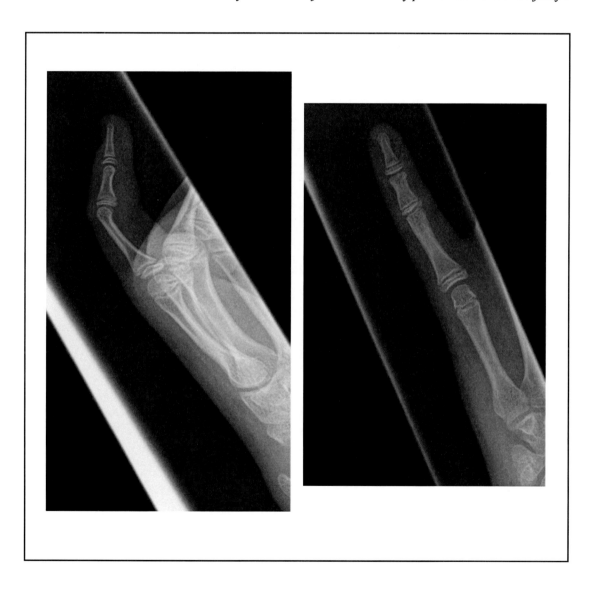

Answer to Case 20

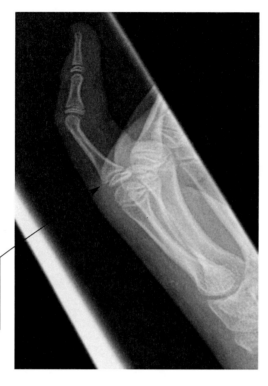

Small Salter Harris type II fracture dorsal aspect of base of proximal phalanx

As demonstrated in the above image, there is a small Salter Harris type II fracture dorsal aspect of the base of the proximal phalanx. This is a difficult area on which to visualise subtle injuries. As previously stated, an oblique view would have been helpful, to avoid the risk of missing subtle injuries.

Hyperextension injuries of the finger often result in avulsion fractures of the volar aspect of the base of the middle phalanx, the so-called volar plate avulsion in adults. In children or adolescents, it is normally a Salter Harris type injury of the volar aspect of the base of the middle phalanx.

Alternatively, a hyperextension injury of the finger may result in a compression injury of the dorsal aspect of the base of the proximal phalanx, as in this case. In a paediatric patient, it may result in a Salter Harris type injury or a torus fracture of the dorsal aspect of the base of the proximal phalanx.

5.

Elbow and forearm trauma

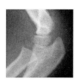

Case 21

Patient fell onto elbow, now not using arm, bony tenderness at elbow area.

Describe the radiograph.

Is there a joint effusion?

What line is useful in assessing this type of injury in children?

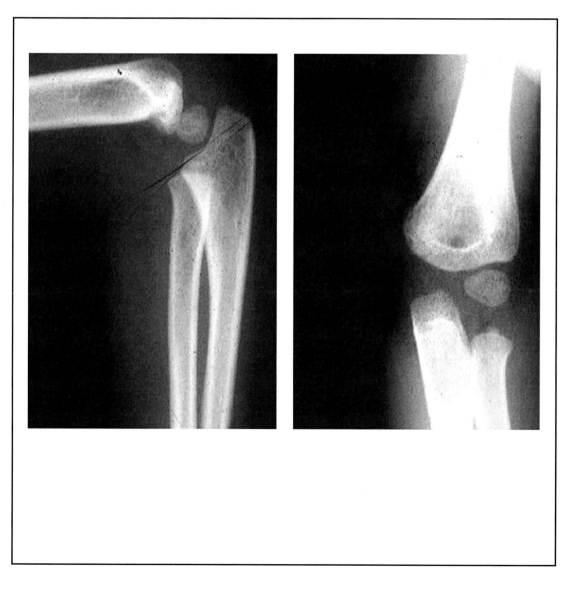

Answer to Case 21

There is a supracondylar fracture. A lucent line and a break in the cortex can be seen at the volar aspect of the distal humeral metaphysis, and the medial epicondyle.

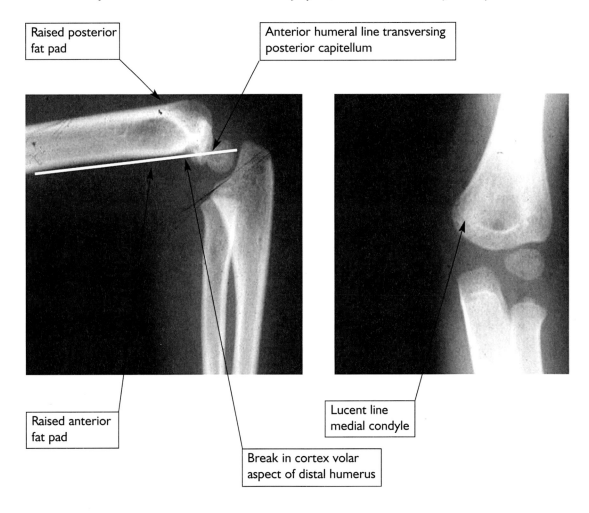

Raised posterior fat pad

Anterior humeral line transversing posterior capitellum

Raised anterior fat pad

Break in cortex volar aspect of distal humerus

Lucent line medial condyle

Sixty per cent of elbow fractures in children are supracondylar fractures. The main mechanism of injury is a fall onto an outstretched hand, although one per cent are caused by a direct fall onto the olecranon. The injury may result in cubitus varus or valgus. Most supracondylar fractures have posterior displacement of the condyles and an abnormal anterior humeral line. The injury may be occult. The main clues to injury are a positive fat pad sign (a joint effusion) and the anterior humeral line not passing through the anterior part of the middle third of the capitellum.

A thin layer of fat lies between the synovial and fibrous layers of both the anterior and posterior aspects of the elbow joint capsule. The two anterior fat pads lie in front of the coronoid fossa and radial fossa of the distal humerus, frequently merged anatomically, and can be seen on the radiograph as a straight lucency making an angle of 30 degrees. The posterior fat pad lies in the intercondylar depression of the posterior surface of the humerus and is not normally demonstrated radiographically. With a small joint effusion an abnormal convex or elevated ('sail sign') anterior fat pad may be seen. With a larger joint effusion the posterior fat pad will also be demonstrated on the lateral radiograph. Remember, though, that if the injury has caused a lot of soft tissue damage and the joint capsule is torn there will be no joint effusion demonstrated radiographically, as the fluid will flow away from the joint.

This case demonstrates a raised anterior fat pad, and posterior fat pad – there is a joint effusion.

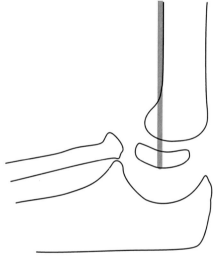

Figure 5.1
Anterior humeral line

The most useful line for demonstrating a supracondylar fracture is the anterior humeral line. If you draw a line along the anterior border of the humerus, on a true lateral radiograph it should bisect the anterior part of the middle third of the capitellum. In this case the anterior humeral line bisects the posterior third of the capitellum which, along with the positive fat pad signs, is indicative of a supracondylar fracture, even if a fracture line cannot be seen. A patient with a positive fat pad sign and an anterior humeral line *not* transversing the correct part of the capitellum, should be treated as a supracondylar fracture, and re-x-rayed 10 to 14 days later, when often the fracture line is visible as bone is reabsorbed along the fracture line. Furthermore, by day 14 an early healing response should be seen in the form of a periosteal reaction.

Remember the fracture may not be complete; it may be a torus, greenstick or even bow fracture.

In this case, the anterior humeral line passes through the posterior capitellum, indicating anterior displacement of the capitellum (a fall on the point of the elbow). It is more usual for the capitellum to be displaced posteriorly in supracondylar or lateral condylar fractures, in which case the anterior humeral line passes anterior to the middle third of the capitellum – as in Case 22 (a fall on outstretched hand).

It is useful at this stage to review the anatomy of the elbow in children. The elbow is made up of three epiphyses – the trochlea, capitellum and proximal radius; and three apophyses – the olecranon, medial and lateral epicondyle.

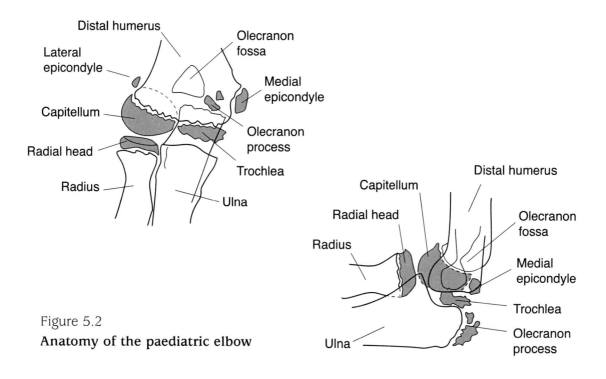

Figure 5.2
Anatomy of the paediatric elbow

As can be seen in the diagram both the olecranon process and trochlea can be quite fragmented, and should not be mistaken as a fracture. The medial epicondyle on the lateral radiograph can sometimes lie quite posteriorly, but should not lie within the joint (see Case 26).

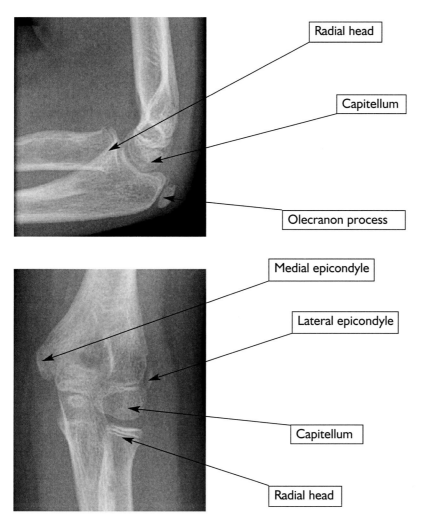

Figure 5.3
Epiphyses and apophyses of the elbow joint

Epiphyses
- Capitellum
- Radial head
- Trochlea

Apophyses
- Lateral epicondyle (origin: common forearm extensor muscles origin)
- Medial epicondyle (origin: common forearm flexor muscle origin)
- Olecranon (insertion: triceps brachii)

91

Case 22

Patient fell on outstretched hand, not using elbow.

Describe the radiographs.

Is there a joint effusion?

Is the anterior humeral line within normal limits?

Is the olecranon normal?

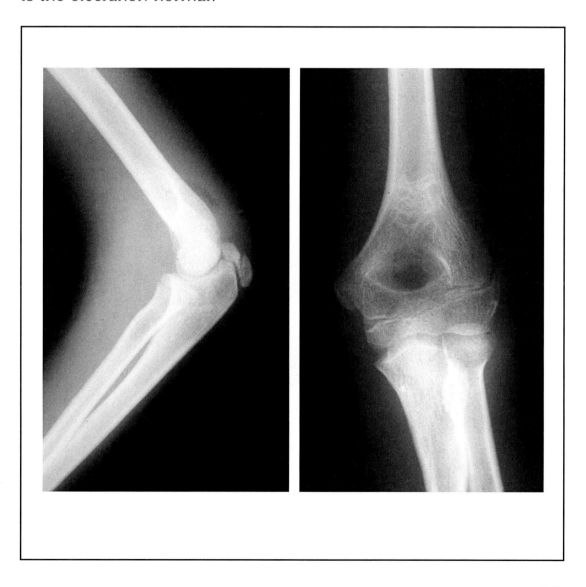

Answer to Case 22

There is a lucent line entering the medial/superior olecranon notch, which is probably a supracondylar fracture. There are positive anterior and posterior fat pads, hence there is a joint effusion. The anterior humeral line traverses the anterior capitellum indicative of a supracondylar fracture. The olecranon process is normal.

The elbow in children is made up of both epiphyses and apophyses (see Figure 5.3). An epiphysis is for longitudinal growth of a bone and is within a joint, an apophysis does not contribute to longitudinal growth of the bone and is not within a joint. Multicentric ossification of these secondary centres may erroneously suggest fragmentation or fracture; the fragmented olecranon process in this case is normal.

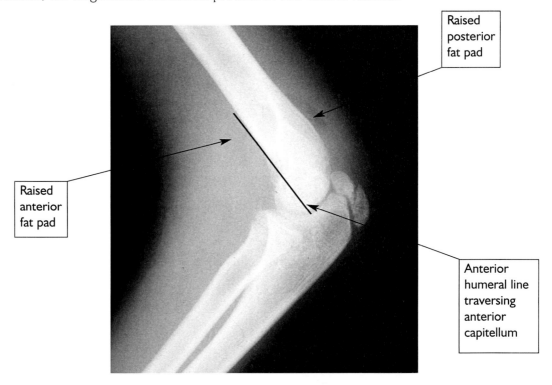

Raised posterior fat pad

Raised anterior fat pad

Anterior humeral line traversing anterior capitellum

The original report for this patient noted the joint effusion and abnormal anterior humeral, commenting that they were indicative of a supracondylar fracture. Hence the patient was treated as a supracondylar fracture and re-x-rayed 14 days later. Now you can see the fracture line (although it was visible on the initial radiographs), and a periosteal reaction along the anterior/medial border of the distal humerus, as it starts to heal.

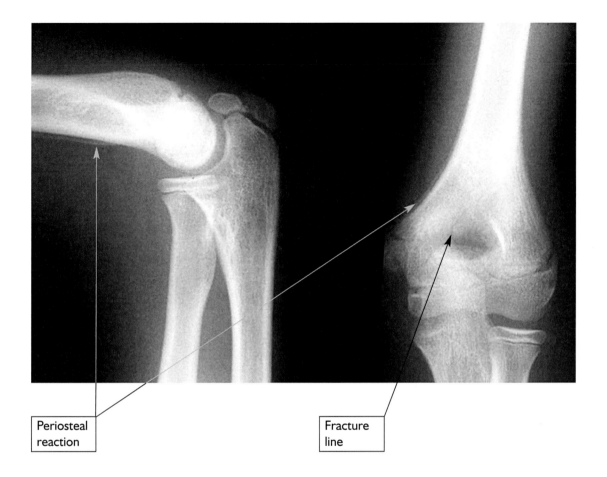

Periosteal
reaction

Fracture
line

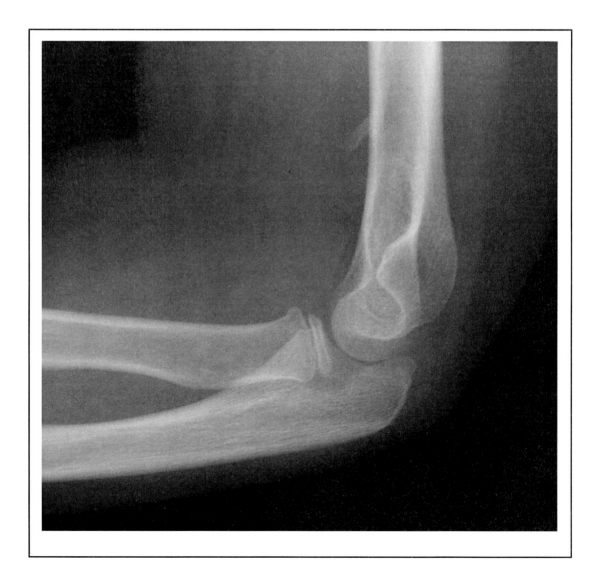

Case 23

Patient fell on outstretched hand. Describe the radiographs (below and on page 96 opposite).

Is there a joint effusion?

Is this a true lateral view?

Is the bony protuberance of the anterior humerus normal? What is it called? Does it have any significance

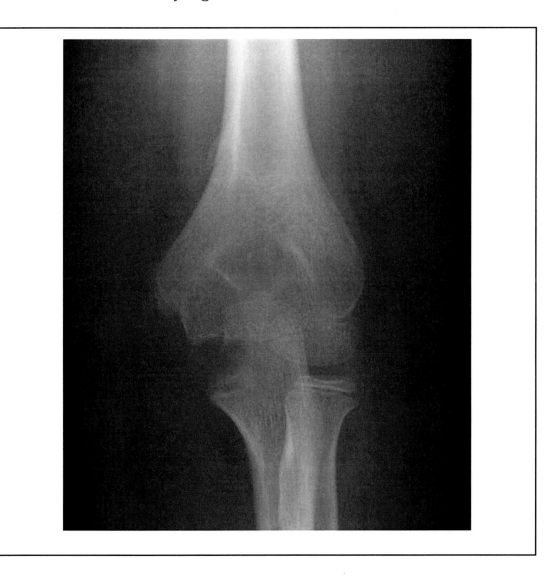

Answer to Case 23

There is a lucent line traversing the superior aspect of the metaphysis of the proximal radius, entering the physeal plate. This is a Salter Harris type II injury. The lateral radiograph is not a true lateral which can make it difficult in the assessment of raised fat pads and affect the anterior humeral line (although in this age group it can be extremely difficult to achieve high-quality radiographs). The lateral radiograph demonstrates a triangular anterior fat pad, which is somewhat raised, but would be more readily demonstrated on a true lateral; posteriorly a fat pad can be visualised overlaid by bone (this would be more readily appreciated on a true lateral). The fracture is radiographically demonstrated and, due to the patient's age, a repeat true lateral radiograph is not required – it would not alter patient management and would increase the child's radiation dose.

The radiograph also demonstrates a bony protuberance on the anterior, medial border of the distal humerus – a supracondylar spur. The supracondylar spur can lie close to the site of the supracondylar fracture, therefore a fracture of the spur may compress or injure either the brachial artery or median nerve.

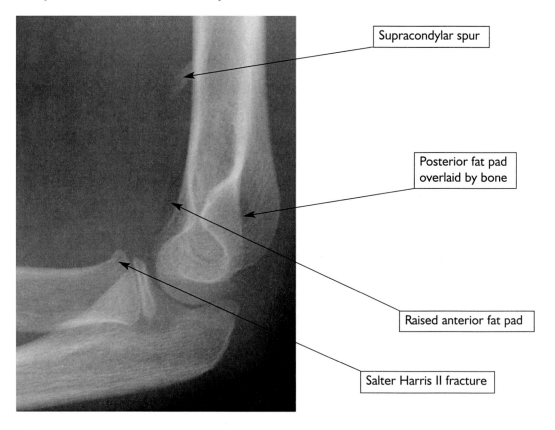

Supracondylar spur

Posterior fat pad overlaid by bone

Raised anterior fat pad

Salter Harris II fracture

Case 24

Patient fell onto arm yesterday, now not using arm and crying on movement.

X-ray request asked for whole arm to be x-rayed.

Describe the radiograph.

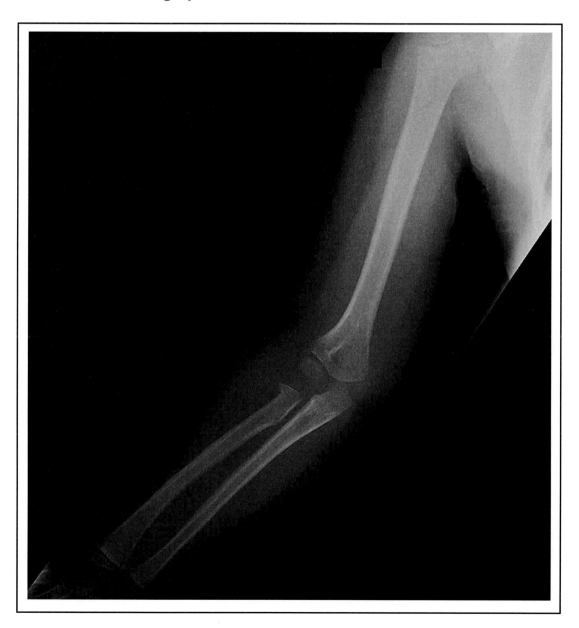

Answer to Case 24

Unfortunately only one radiograph is available. Depending on the age and size of the child we should always obtain separate arm and forearm radiographs, otherwise subtle fractures may be missed. This radiograph demonstrates a transverse fracture of the radial head, an unusual injury in this age group (see Case 1). This case reminds us that the associations between injury type and age groups (see p. 41) are just guidelines to help in radiological diagnosis.

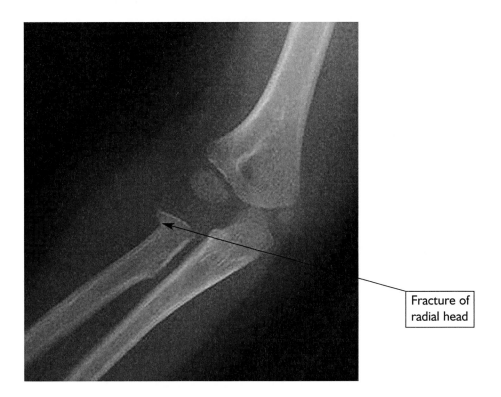

Fracture of radial head

Case 25

Patient fell onto arm, now painful whole length of forearm, with limited movement.

Describe the radiographs.

Would another view be helpful?

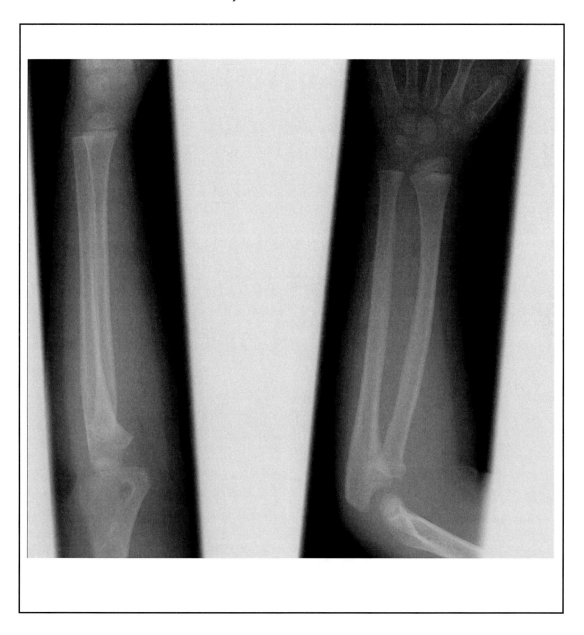

Answer to Case 25

A positive anterior fat pad can be seen at the elbow and there appears to be a buckle fracture of the volar aspect of the radial head. This demonstrates the importance of looking carefully at all aspects of the radiograph, particularly the edges. An anterior posterior radiograph of the elbow would be useful; because the radiograph was taken to demonstrate the forearm, an oblique presentation of the elbow joint has been obtained. The anterior posterior view demonstrates the fracture and steep radial angulation (about 45 degrees) of the metaphysis.

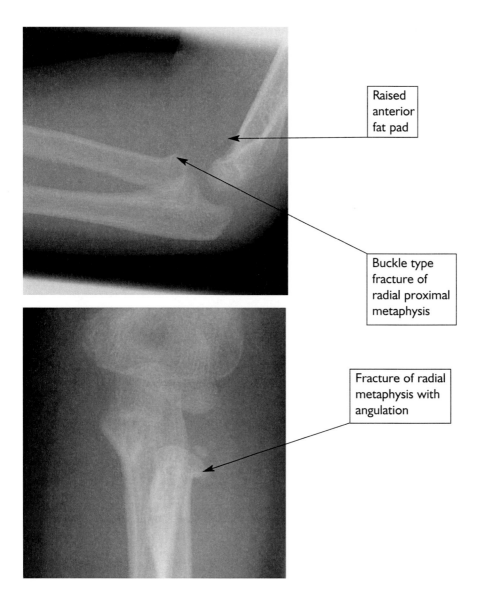

Raised anterior fat pad

Buckle type fracture of radial proximal metaphysis

Fracture of radial metaphysis with angulation

Case 26

Adolescent fell, injuring elbow; unsure of mechanism of injury.

Describe the radiograph.

What is the normal mechanism of injury for this type of trauma?

What complication can occur in this type of injury?

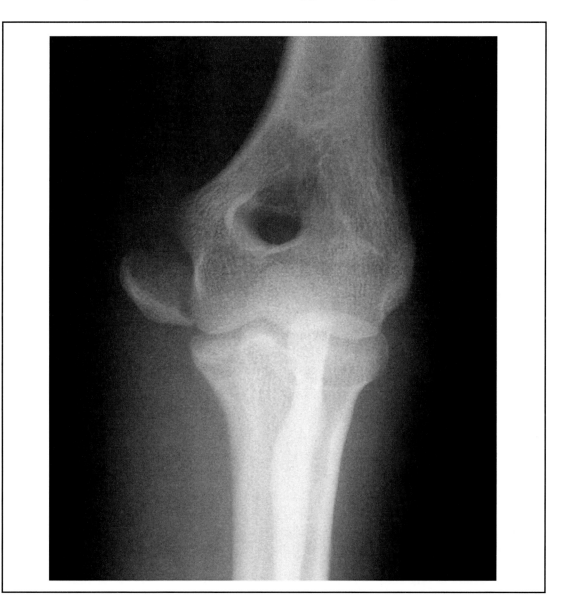

Answer to Case 26

This is an older child, where the physeal plates have fused. There is an avulsion of the medial epicondyle. Ten per cent of elbow injuries in children are avulsions of the medial epicondyle. Mechanisms of injury are a fall on the outstretched hand, violent contraction of the flexor pronator muscle during the act of throwing (sometimes called 'little leaguer's elbow', in America), or dislocation of the elbow.

One of the complications that can occur is entrapment of the medial epicondyle (occurs in ten per cent of children) but this may go unrecognised, resulting in severe late disability. Valgus stress initially occurs at the time of injury with temporary widening of the elbow joint space medially. The avulsed epicondyle is drawn into the joint by traction from the attached flexor pronator muscle group, and the ulnar collateral ligament. When the force is released the joint is closed, entrapping the medial epicondyle. Prior to the appearance of all the epiphyses and apophyses the injury may go unrecognised as the avulsed epicondyle is mistaken for the trochlea. It is therefore important to know the ossification sequence of the elbow.

There are two memory aids, the most common being the acronym **CRITOL**.

- **C** apitellum – 1 year

- **R** adial head – 3 to 6 years

- **I** nternal (medial) epicondyle – 4 to 7 years

- **T** rochlea – 9 to 10 years

- **O** lecranon – 10 years

- **L** ateral epicondyle – 11 years

Hence the trochlea is never seen radiographically without also seeing the medial epicondyle.

An alternative for remembering the sequence of ossification of the elbow is Nelson's X mnemonic, as demonstrated in Figure 5.4.

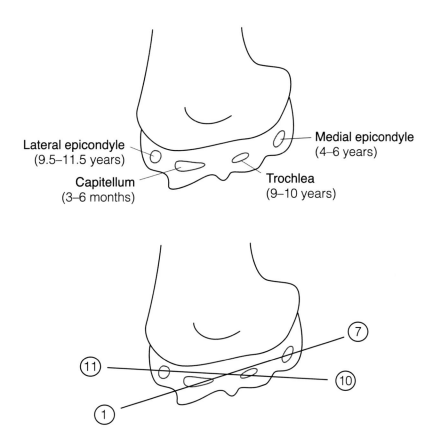

Figure 5.4
Nelson's X mnemonic for sequence of ossification of the elbow – 1, 7, 10, 11 (years)

Avulsions of the medial epicondyle may be subtle, and there are not always positive fat pads as a clue to injury, because the medial epicondyle is extracapsular in some patients. Also when associated with dislocation the joint capsule may be disrupted, allowing escape of joint fluids. The medial epicondyle may lie quite posteriorly on the lateral radiograph (see Case 21); it should not however project over the region of the capitellum or joint space. When reviewing a radiograph for avulsion of the medial epicondyle look for loss of parallelism between the epicondyle and adjacent metaphysis. The medial apophyseal centre should have a complete surrounding thin rim of sclerosis; with subtle malrotations subsequent to fracture this peripheral rim may be absent.

Case 27

Patient fell injuring elbow, now painful, with limited movement.

Describe the radiographs.

Following this type of injury, what other area of the arm should be radiographically reviewed?

What is the name of the normal variant demonstrated?

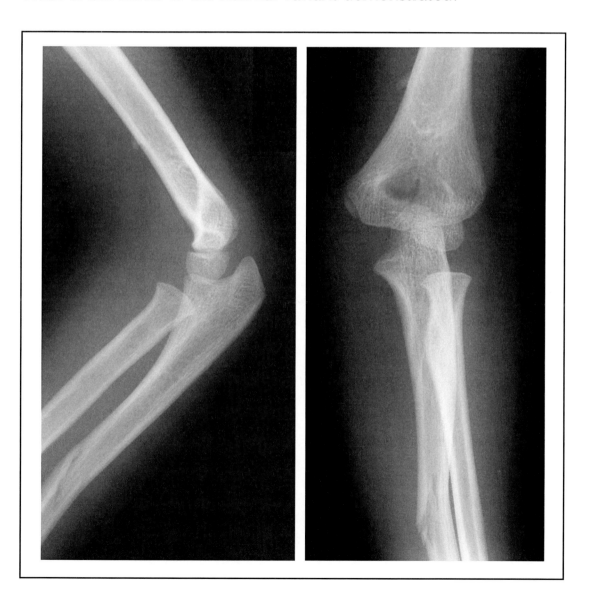

Answer to Case 27

There is a greenstick type fracture of the mid third of the ulna. The radius and ulna are like a bony ring – if you identify a fracture of one then look for a fracture of the other or for a dislocation. The whole length of the radius and ulna including the elbow and wrist joints needs to be radiographed. There is no fracture of the radius in this case (demonstrated on the radiographs that follow). If only the ulna is fractured then look carefully at the radial head, and use the radiocapitellar line to check for dislocation (an ulnar shaft fracture in the presence of a dislocation is termed a Monteggia fracture dislocation). A line drawn along the long axis of the radius should bisect the capitellum (and is not dependent on radiographic position); if it does not then there is dislocation of the radial head.

It is possible to have an isolated fracture of the ulna or radius with no associated dislocation, commonly occuring following a direct blow. An isolated fracture of the ulna is frequently called a 'night stick' injury, occurring when the individual extends an arm up to protect themselves from attack from a 'stick'.

A fracture of the radius associated with dislocation at the radio–ulnar joint, is called a Galeazzi fracture dislocation. With a Monteggia fracture dislocation in an adult the fracture is often obvious, the dislocation of the radial head less so; in children the fracture is often less obvious, as it may be an incomplete fracture. There is no dislocation of the radial head in this case; it is not a Monteggia fracture dislocation.

The normal variant demonstrated in this case is a supracondylar spur (see Case 23).

Table 5.1 **Monteggia fracture dislocation in children**

Type	Dislocation of radial head	Ulnar fracture	Radial fracture
I (most common)	Anterior	Proximal 1/3 of shaft, anterior angulation	
II	Posterior	Proximal 1/3 of shaft, posterior angulation	
III (second most common associated with radial neck injury)	Lateral	Metaphyseal (greenstick)	
IV	Anterior	Proximal 1/3 of shaft	Proximal radius

Monteggia equivalent type fracture equals fracture of the proximal radius without radial head dislocation.

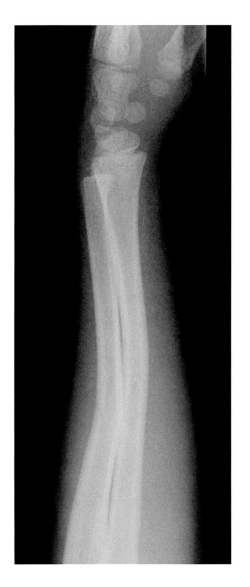
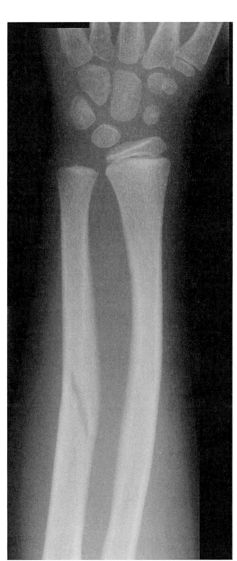

Case 28

Patient fell whilst doing a handstand, now painful forearm.

Describe the radiographs.

What is the name for this type of injury?

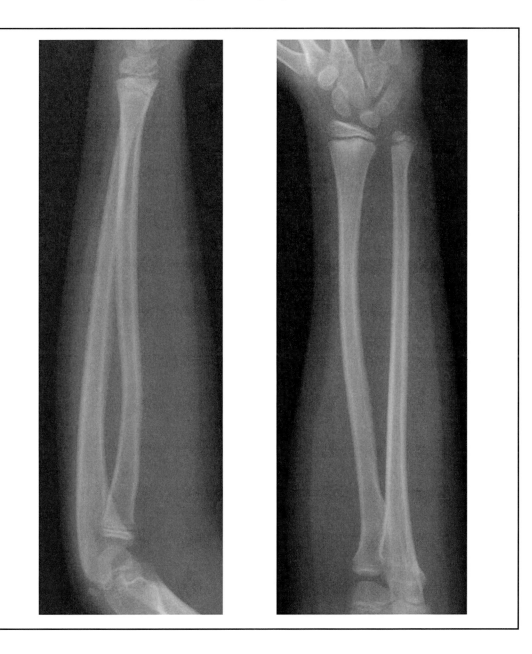

Answer to Case 28

There is a greenstick fracture (a subtle break in cortex at the site of angulation) of the proximal radius. Distally there is loss of congruity at the radio–ulnar joint. This is called a Galeazzi fracture dislocation. As mentioned in Case 27 the forearm should be treated as a bony ring; if one fracture is identified, look for another or a dislocation. The ulna normally lies two millimetres proximal to the distal radius; remember that there are ulnar variances – both negative and positive variants. Ulnar negative variance is associated with Keinboch's disease (avascular necrosis of the lunate). Ulnar positive variance is associated with increased incidence of triangular fibrocartilage tears.

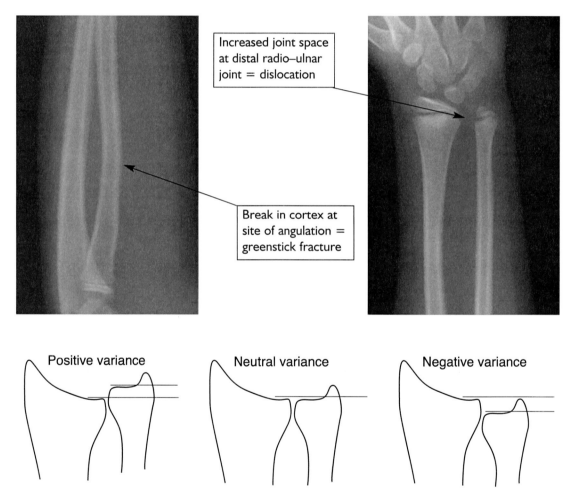

Increased joint space at distal radio–ulnar joint = dislocation

Break in cortex at site of angulation = greenstick fracture

Positive variance   Neutral variance   Negative variance

Figure 5.5 **Ulnar variance (true dorsipalmar radiograph required with no rotation)**
Normal range = 2.3 to 4.2 cm

Case 29

Patient fell during games, unsure of mechanism of injury. All forearm painful, difficulty moving arm.

Describe the radiographs.

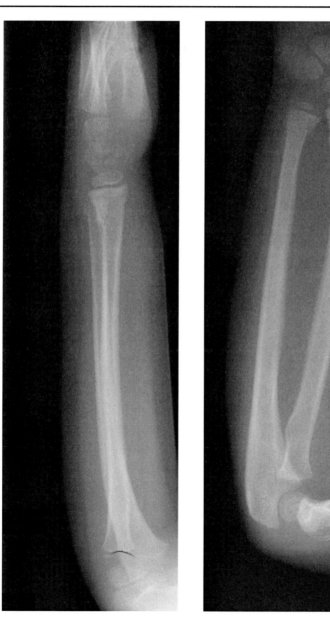

Answer to Case 29

There is a torus fracture of the distal radius (remember always to look extra carefully at both joints on forearm radiographs). In adults a number of patients that have fracture of the distal radius also have fractures of the distal ulna; this is also the case in children, hence the distal ulna requires careful review. The anterior posterior radiograph demonstrates what appears to be a greenstick fracture of the distal ulna. On review of the lateral radiograph a completely separated fragment of the dorsal aspect of the ulnar metaphysis is demonstrated, a Salter Harris II type injury. Also demonstrated on the lateral view is the dorsal angulation of the distal radius (remember the distal radius is normally angulated volarly by 10 to 15 degrees).

Case 30

Patient fell onto arm, painful forearm, unable to move arm.

Describe the radiographs.

What is this type of injury called?

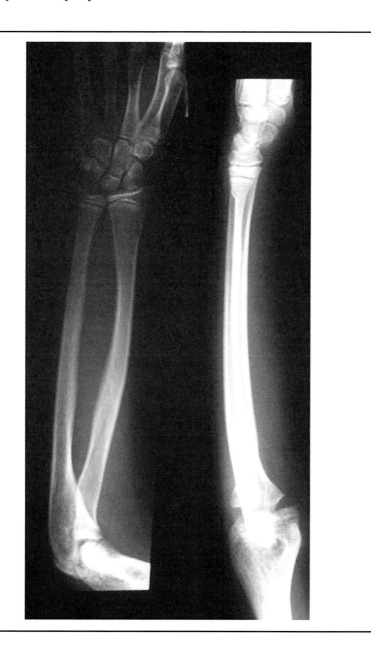

Answer to Case 30

The lateral radiograph demonstrates a torus fracture of the dorsal aspect of the distal radial metaphysis, a common injury from a fall on the outstretched hand. This case highlights the importance of looking carefully at all aspects of the forearm, particularly both joints.

Case 31

Patient fell from bicycle onto elbow, now painful with limited range of movement.

Write a provisional image evaluation.

Should other views be considered?

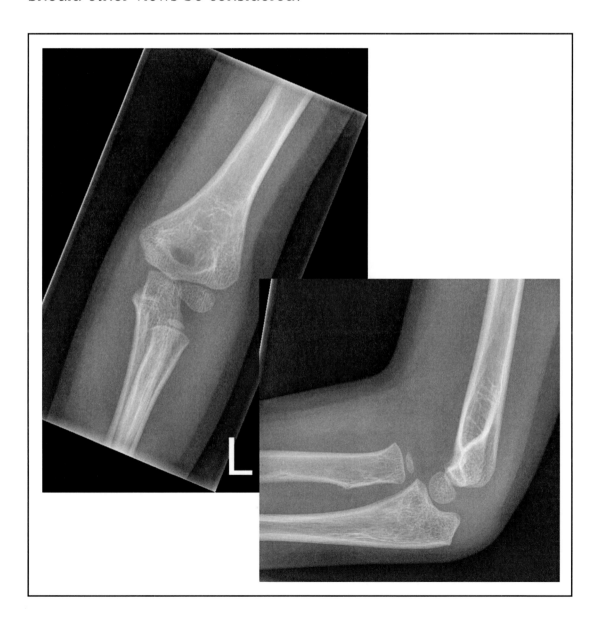

Answer to Case 31

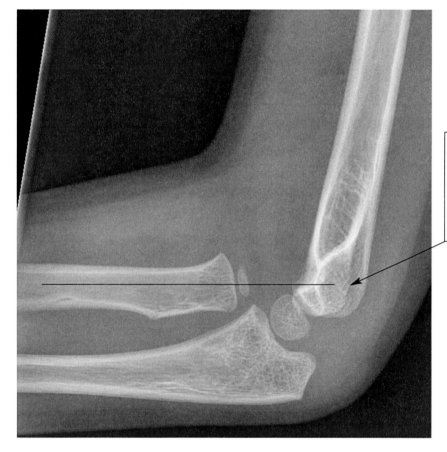

Radio capitellum line does not pass through the capitellum; hence there is a radial head dislocation

The radio capitellum line (which should always be used when reviewing elbow images) does not pass through the capitellum. This means there is a dislocation of the radial head; in this case, a volar dislocation of the radial head. There is also a joint effusion present; in this case, a raised anterior fat pad. Radial head dislocations are associated with fractures of the ulnar, the so-called Monteggia fracture dislocation.

These associated fractures of the ulna are normally just distal to the elbow joint. In children, they can be extremely subtle, as they will probably be incomplete fractures. To conclude, full-length radius and ulnar views should be carried out, to avoid the risk of missing a Monteggia fracture dislocation.

Case 32

Patient fell onto outstretched hand. Now painful elbow, unable to flex, extend, pronate and supinate.

Write a provisional image evaluation.

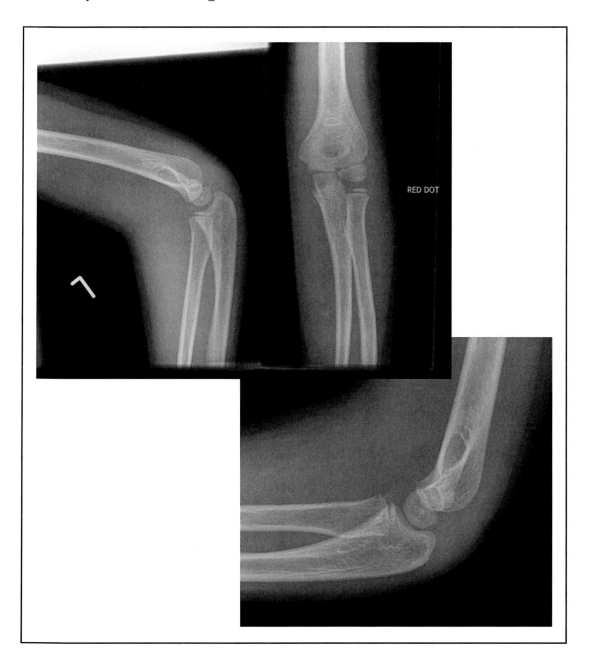

Answer to Case 32

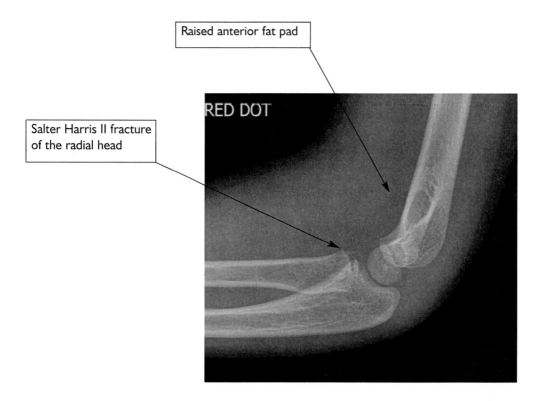

Raised anterior fat pad

Salter Harris II fracture of the radial head

RED DOT

There is a raised anterior fat pad, a joint effusion. This, along with the clinical details, makes one suspicious of a radial head fracture. The most common type of radial head fracture in this age group would be a Salter Harris II fracture of the volar aspect of the radial head; and the repeat lateral view does indeed demonstrate a Salter Harris II fracture of the volar aspect of the radial head.

Case 33

Fell from climbing frame, unable to move elbow.

Write a provisional image evaluation.

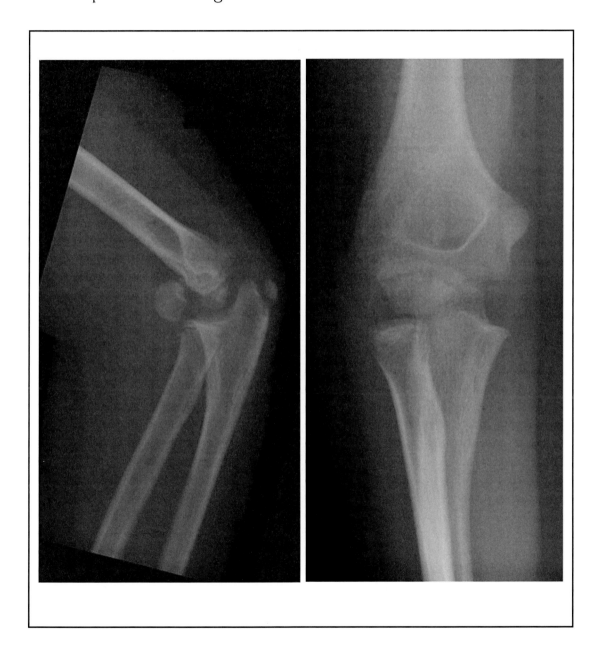

Answer to Case 33

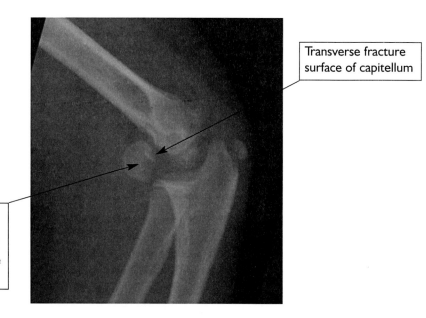

Transverse fracture surface of capitellum

Articular surface of capitellum, no longer articulating with radial head; hence a fracture dislocation

There is a fracture dislocation of the capitellum. As in adults, the transverse fracture of the base of the capitellum has resulted in a 90-degree volar rotation of the capitellum. This means that the articular surface of the capitellum is no longer in apposition with the radial head, resulting in a fracture dislocation. The fracture dislocation of the capitellum can also be visualised on the AP in this case, although this injury is often difficult to visualise on the AP view.

Case 34

Fell onto outstretched hand, now painful elbow with limited movement.

Write a preliminary image evaluation.

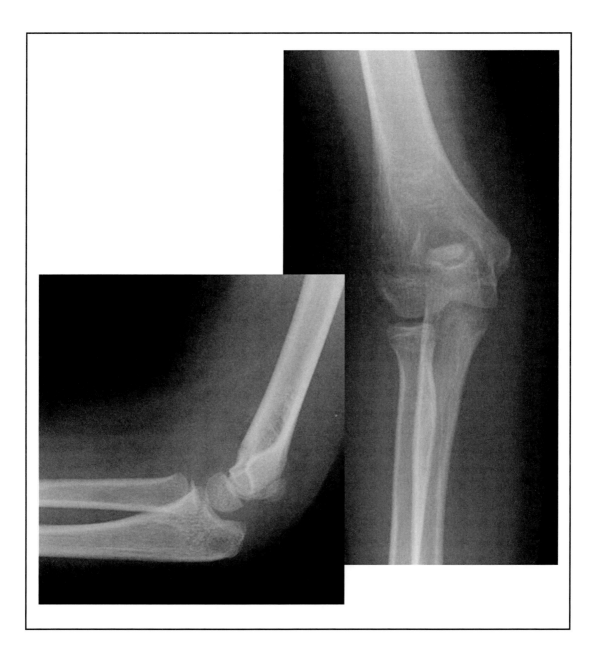

Answer to Case 34

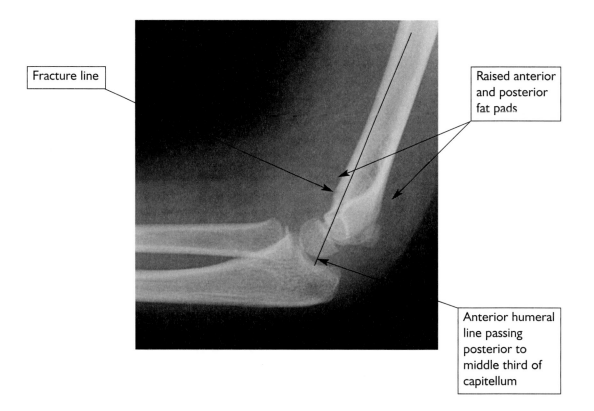

Fracture line

Raised anterior and posterior fat pads

Anterior humeral line passing posterior to middle third of capitellum

This is a subtle supracondylar fracture. There is a large joint effusion (raised anterior and posterior fat pads), with anterior humeral line not passing through anterior part of middle third of capitellum; both these signs indicate a supracondylar fracture. The fracture can actually be visualised on the lateral view.

Case 35

Fell from slide, painful all through forearm, difficult to assess due to pain.

Write a provisional image evaluation.

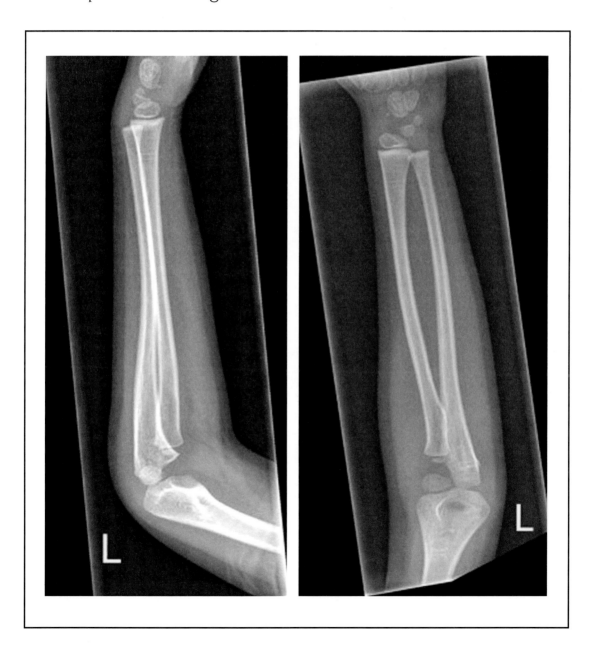

Answer to Case 35

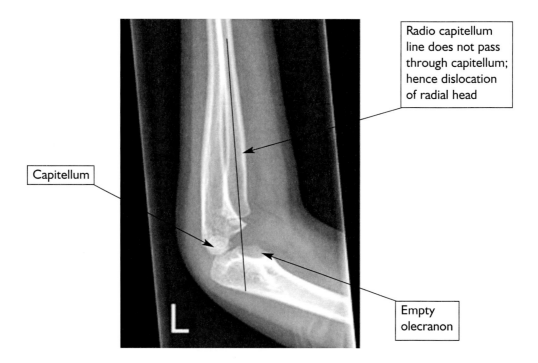

Radio capitellum line does not pass through capitellum; hence dislocation of radial head

Capitellum

Empty olecranon

There is an anterior dislocation of the radial head and proximal olecranon. Even though the images are not perfect, the radio capitellum line does not pass through the capitellum, and the olecranon notch is visibly empty. No definite fracture of the ulna was identified. This demonstrates the importance of looking at all four corners of the image.

6.

Shoulder trauma

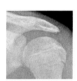

Case 36

Patient fell directly onto shoulder, now painful clavicle on movement.

Describe the radiograph.

What are the main mechanisms of injury?

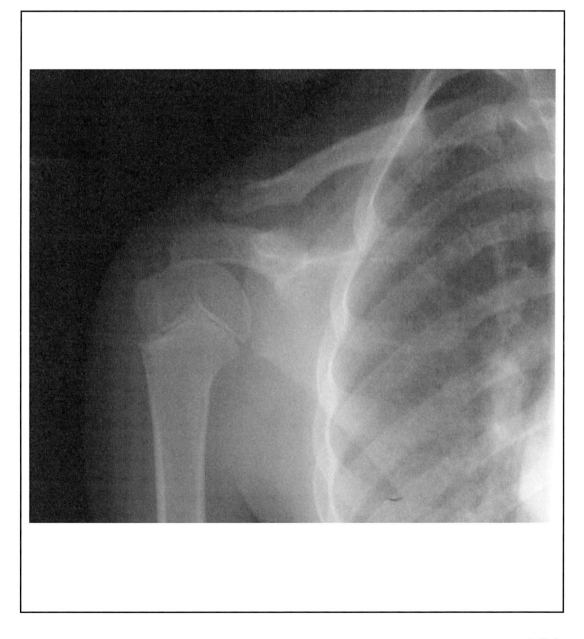

Answer to Case 36

There is a fracture of the distal clavicle. A fracture of the clavicle is common injury in children. Fifty per cent of fractures of the clavicle occur in those under 10 years of age. 90 per cent of fractures of the clavicle are caused by a fall directly onto the shoulder. A direct blow or fall on the outstretched hand are less common mechanisms of injury. Around 80 per cent of fractures occur in the mid clavicle, 15 per cent to the distal clavicle and 5 per cent to the proximal clavicle.

Fractured clavicle

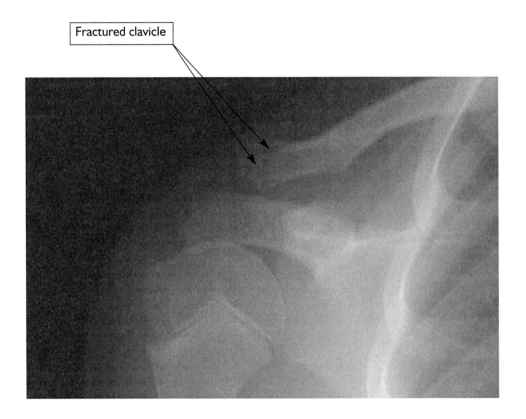

Case 37

Patient fell onto shoulder, now painful at acromio–clavicular joint and length of clavicle.

Describe the radiograph.

Is there an injury?

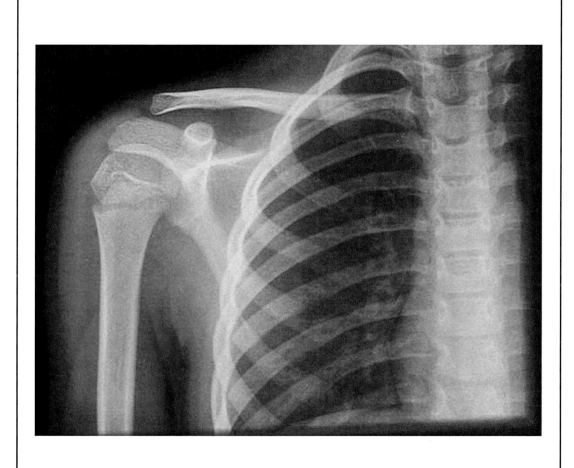

Answer to Case 37

There is no bony injury, or acromio–clavicular joint dislocation demonstrated on these radiographs. The non-alignment of the inferior surface of the acromion and clavicle is normal for a child, but in an adult would represent subluxation. The relative positions of the acromion and clavicle can not be assessed due to unossified cartilage. Acromio–clavicular joint subluxations are rare in children, the normal age range for this injury being 15 to 40 years. However, pseudo dislocation is possible.

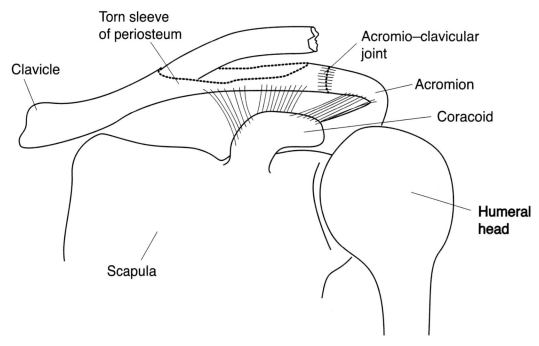

Figure 6.1
Pseudo dislocation of the acromio–clavicular joint in a child

Clinically and radiographically acromio–clavicular pseudo dislocation appears as a complete acromio–clavicular joint dislocation, but at surgery a torn periosteal sleeve is found with intact coraco–clavicular ligaments. If this injury remains untreated a Y-shaped clavicle results.

Case 38

Patient fell directly onto shoulder, now unable to move arm, bony tenderness to clavicle.

Describe the radiograph.

At what age does the medial clavicular epiphysis ossify and fuse?

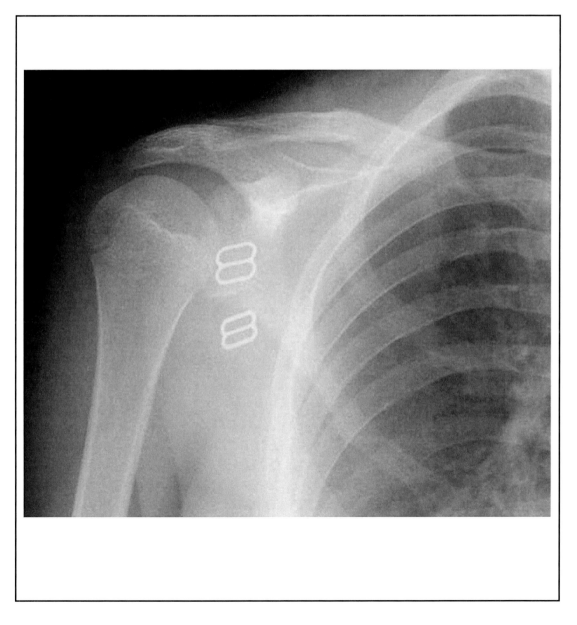

Answer to Case 38

There is a fracture of the mid third of the clavicle (the most common area of the clavicle to fracture). Sometimes this type of fracture can be quite difficult to see as it is often superimposed radiographically over the spine of the scapula. Often when a clavicle fracture is clinically suspected, but not radiographically demonstrated, a cranially angulated radiograph of the clavicle is done (demonstrating it clear of the spine of the scapula).

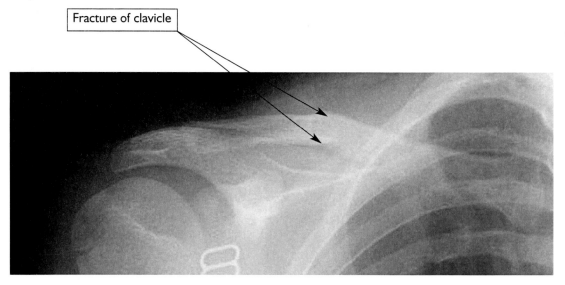

Fracture of clavicle

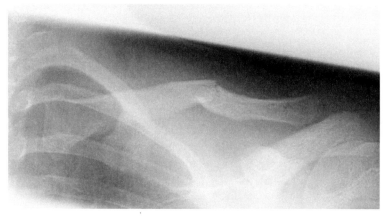

Another case with a cranially angled view of the clavicle demonstrating a mid shaft fracture clear of the spine of scapula.

The medial clavicular epiphysis is the last to ossify, at 18 to 20 years of age, and is the last to fuse, at 25 to 26 years of age. Without this information it is easy to mistake a normal medial clavicle epiphysis as a fracture of the medial clavicle. Hence it is possible to have a Salter Harris I fracture of the medial clavicle up to 26 years of age.

Case 39

Patient fell off slide injuring shoulder, now painful to move.

Describe the radiograph.

How many centres of ossification form the humeral head, and at what age do they appear?

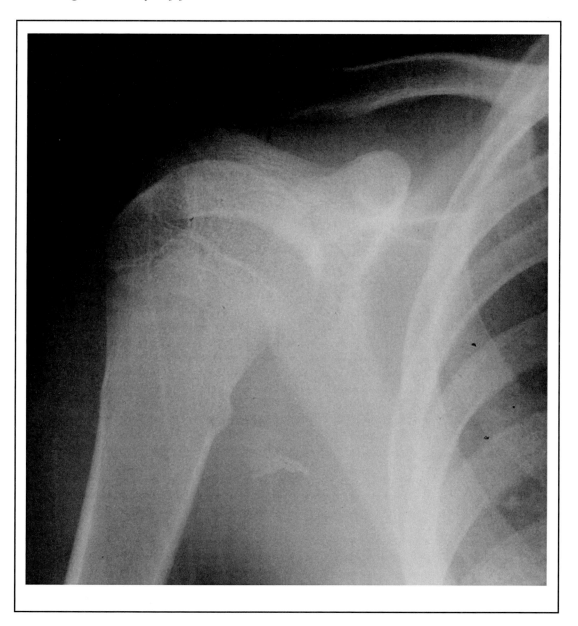

Answer to Case 39

There is a torus fracture of the proximal shaft of the humerus.

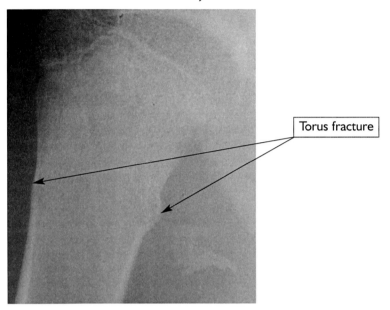

Torus fracture

The humeral head has three centres of ossification. The ossification centre for the humeral head appears first at 4 to 6 months of age, then the greater tubercle at 3 years of age, and the lesser tubercle at 5 years of age; they coalesce at 7 years of age. It is particularly important with children to know what is normal radiographic anatomy so that abnormal anatomy can be more readily identified. It is useful to have a text of normal radiographic anatomy at different ages at hand for the radiograph reporter. Below are three normal radiographs at different ages of the shoulder to give an idea of the normal radiographic anatomy, when the humeral head ossification centres appear.

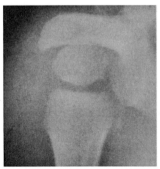 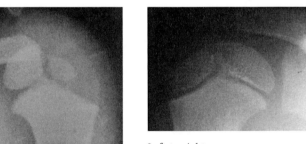

Left to right
4–6 months to 3 years
3 to 5 years
5 years until fusion

Figure 6.2
Normal shoulder radiographs in children

Case 40

Patient fell onto shoulder, bony tenderness to humeral head.

Describe the radiographs.

Classify the injury.

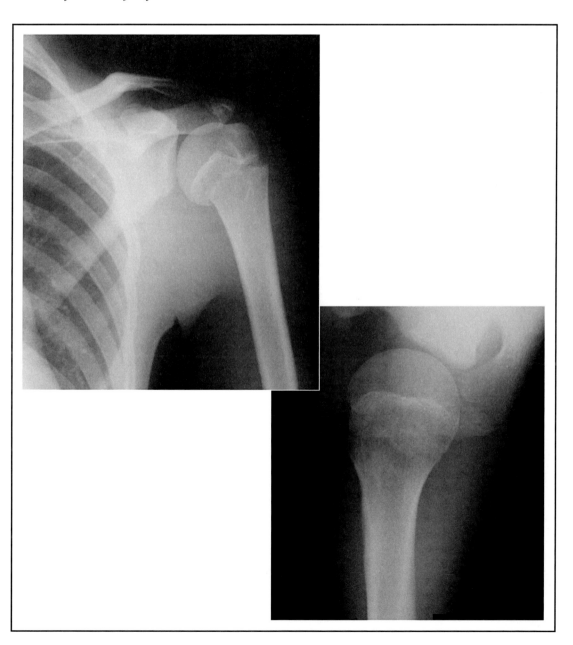

Answer to Case 40

There is a separation of the humeral head physeal plate lateral aspect (anteroposterior radiograph), involving the metaphysis medially (axial radiograph); this is a Salter Harris type II injury. There is lateral displacement of the diaphysis (remember always describe movement of the distal part, not the proximal part).

The proximal humeral physeal plate on the anterior posterior view in external rotation is shaped like an inverted V or chevron. Below shows a normal humeral physeal plate – care is needed not to mistake the physeal plate for a fracture. The proximal humeral epiphysis is responsible for 80 per cent of growth of the humerus. Physeal separation is rare, but most commonly occurs from 10 to 15 years of age. Salter Harris I injuries are more common in the under 10s, whereas Salter Harris II are more common in the 10–15 age group.

Normal physeal plate of humerus

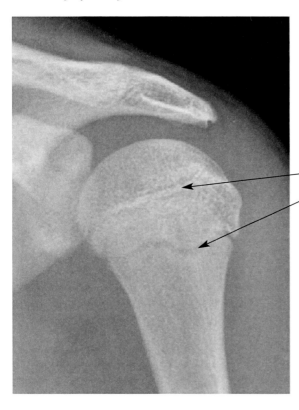

Normal double line of physis (if you follow one round it will join up with the other) – not to be mistaken as a fracture

Case 41

Patient fell hitting proximal humerus against a shelf, now extremely painful.

Describe the radiograph.

Name the pathology.

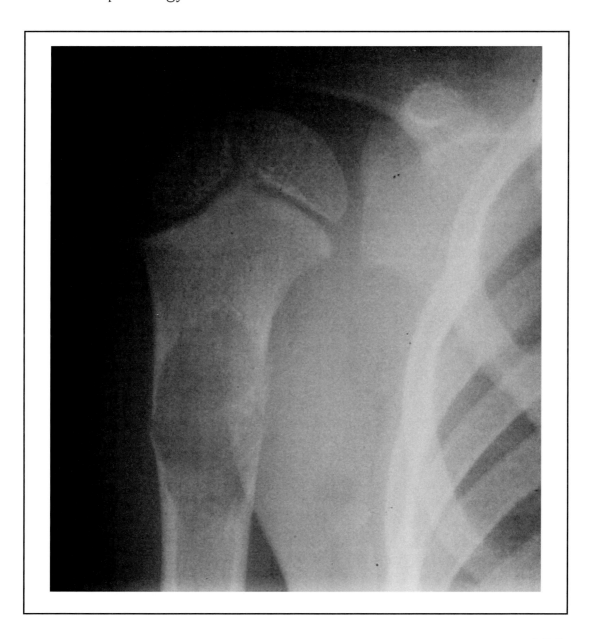

Answer to Case 41

There is a fracture through a simple bone cyst in the proximal humeral diaphysis. No lateral radiograph was available.

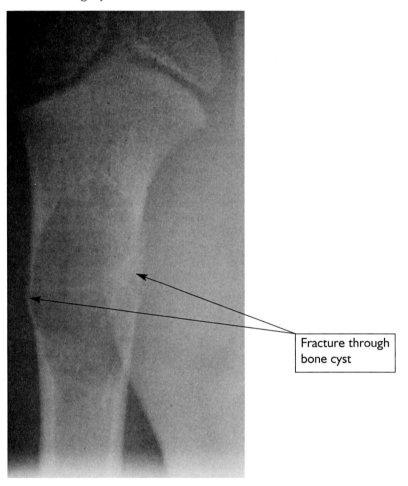

Fracture through bone cyst

This is a benign fluid-filled bone lesion of children (sometimes called a unicameral bone cyst). These cysts are often central geographic lesions, often in the metaphysis, but may migrate to the diaphysis (as in this case) as the skeleton matures. Proximal humerus is the most common site (50 per cent), although sometimes they occur in the proximal femur (20 per cent). Occasionally they may heal spontaneously following fracture.

Case 42

Fourteen-year-old patient fell onto shoulder, painful acromion.

Describe the radiograph.

At what age do the coracoid and acromion apophyses fuse?

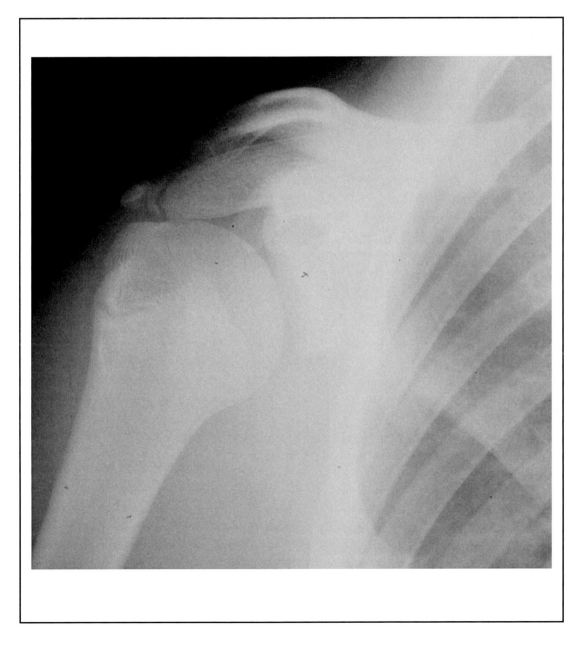

Answer to Case 42

There is no bony injury. The lucency seen crossing the lateral tip of the acromion is an apophysis. If you look carefully the coracoid apophysis can also be seen. The scapula arises from several ossification centres that can easily be mistaken for fractures. Small slivers of ossification centres on the superior aspect of coracoid and the acromion can easily be mistaken for avulsion fractures. The coracoid and acromion apophyses fuse at about 15 years of age; the apophysis of the inferior border of the scapula fuses at about 20 years of age.

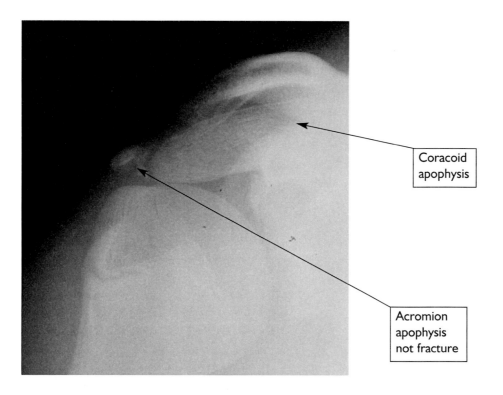

Coracoid apophysis

Acromion apophysis not fracture

Case 43

Patient fell off swing, limited movement in shoulder.

Describe the radiographs.

Where are the physeal plate, metaphysis and diaphysis of the humerus?

Where are the glenoid, acromion and coracoid on the axial view?

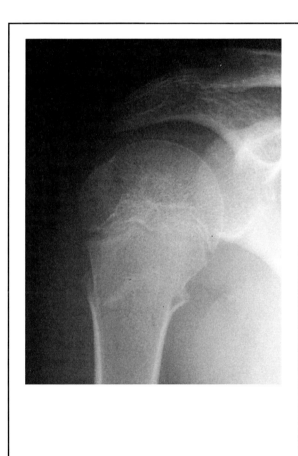
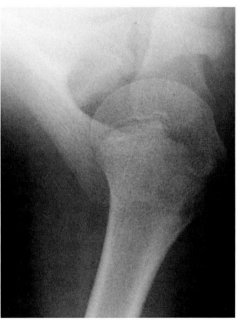

Answer to Case 43

There is a fracture of the surgical neck of the humerus. When reviewing children's shoulder radiographs take care not to mistake the physeal plate of the humerus for a fracture. Often two physeal lines can be seen (as shown below), but if you trace one of the physeal lines round it should meet up with the other physeal line (see Case 40). The epiphysis, metaphysis and diaphysis are shown in the anterior posterior radiograph.

Anterior posterior radiograph

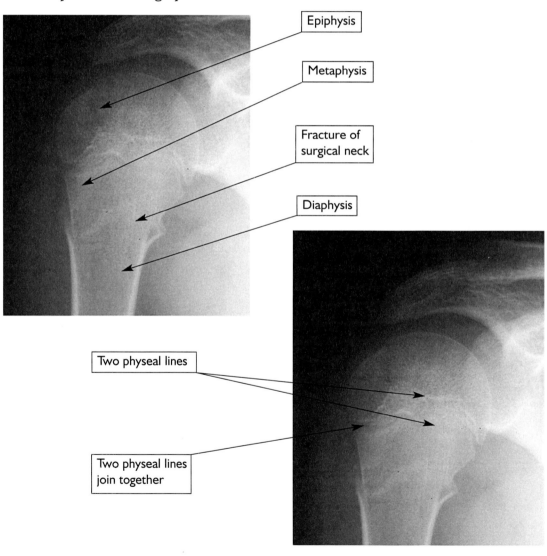

The acromion, glenoid fossa and coracoid are seen in the axial view.

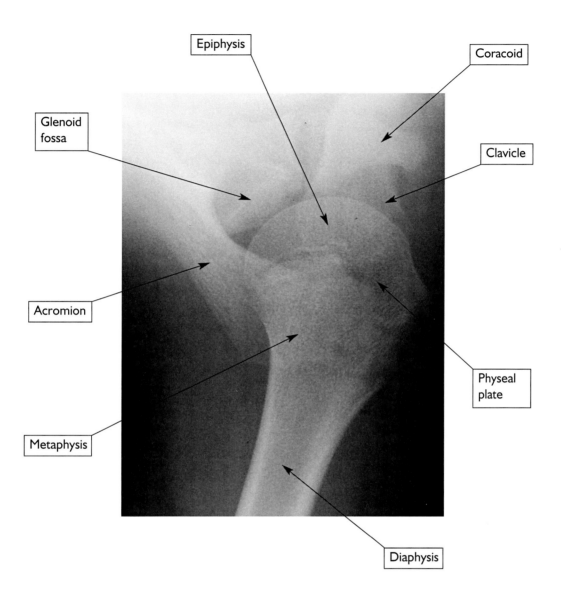

Case 44

Patient fell from bike onto shoulder, now limited movement.

Describe the radiographs.

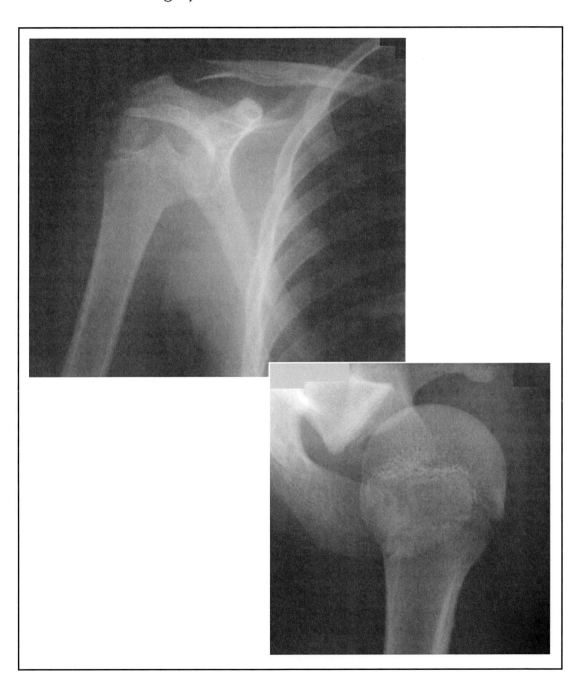

Answer to Case 44

There is a sudden angulation at the medial aspect of the surgical neck of the humerus (demonstrated on the anterior posterior view), which is indicative of a fracture. The axial view clearly demonstrates a break in the cortex which appears to cross the shaft of the bone. This lucent line is not a physeal plate but a fracture (it does not join up with the physeal line seen proximal to it; see Cases 40 and 43).

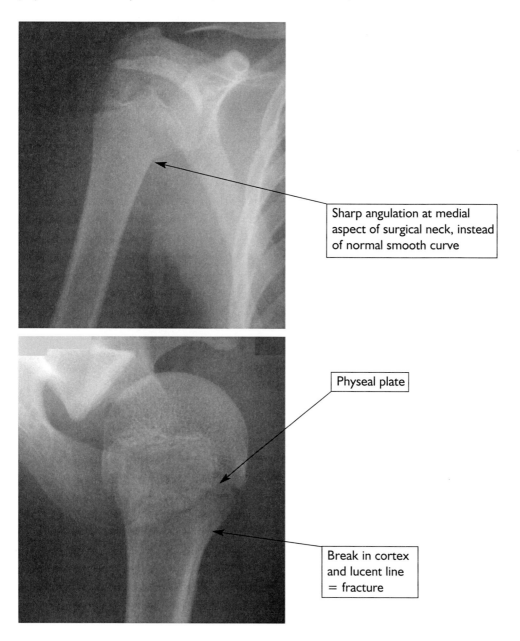

Sharp angulation at medial aspect of surgical neck, instead of normal smooth curve

Physeal plate

Break in cortex and lucent line = fracture

Case 45

Patient suffered from previous dislocations and subluxations of the shoulder. Today painful shoulder following playing football.

Describe the radiographs.

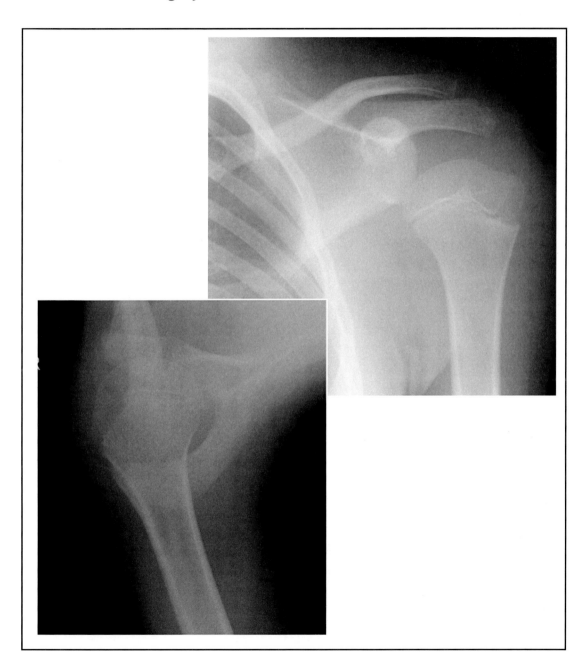

Answer to Case 45

The anterior posterior radiograph demonstrates that the humeral head has moved inferiorly with regards to the glenoid. The axial view demonstrates that the articular surface of the humeral head is no longer in apposition with the glenoid – it is an anterior dislocation of the humeral head. Dislocations are relatively rare in children, but as with adults always require two projections (an anterior posterior view and an axial, or Y view or modified axial) to assess whether there is a dislocation.

Modified axial view

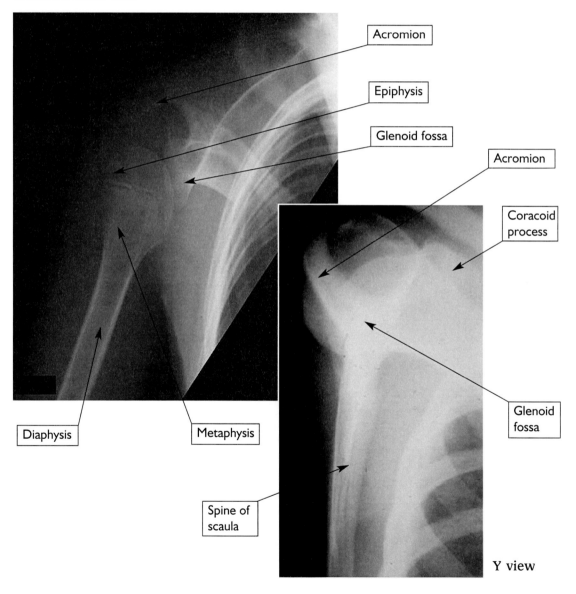

Acromion

Epiphysis

Glenoid fossa

Acromion

Coracoid process

Diaphysis

Metaphysis

Glenoid fossa

Spine of scaula

Y view

7.

Ankle and foot trauma

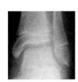

Case 46

Patient fell off skateboard, injuring ankle.

Describe the radiographs.

Classify the injury.

Comment on the age that the ankle ossification centres appear.

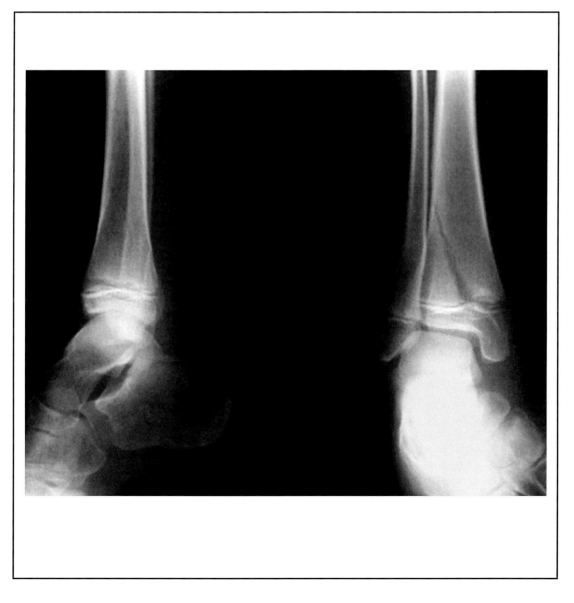

Answer to Case 46

There is an oblique fracture of the distal tibia entering the physeal plate (resulting in widening of the physeal plate medially); there is also a small fragment of bone in the medial physeal plate. Any fracture that involves the physeal plate can be classified using the Salter Harris classification system. This is a Salter Harris type II injury (see Figure 2.4 p. 00). There is also a torus injury of the distal fibula diaphysis.

Ossification centres of the ankle joint

- 6 months – distal tibial epiphysis appears

- 18 months – distal fibular epiphysis appears

- 5 years – epiphysis same width as metaphysis

- 10 years – malleoli well developed

- 12–13 years – assume adult appearance, fusion begins

- 14 years – tibia fused (girls), fibula 1 year later (boys fuse later)

On the next page are some ankle radiographs at various developmental stages, to assist when differentiating the normal ankle radiograph from the abnormal – as mentioned previously it is vital to have readily available texts of normal development and variants.

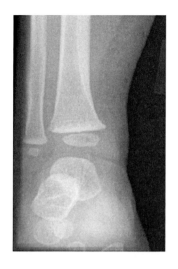
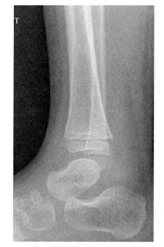

Normal epiphysis at 1 year

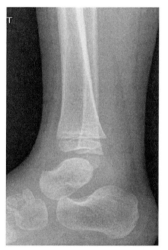
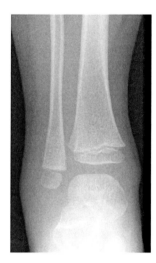

Normal epiphysis at 4 years

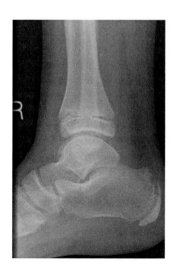
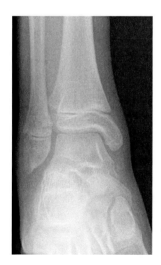

Normal epiphysis at 12 years

Case 47

Patient fell twisting ankle, now bony tenderness of distal tibia and fibula.

Describe the radiographs.

Discuss the use of additional radiographs in this patient.

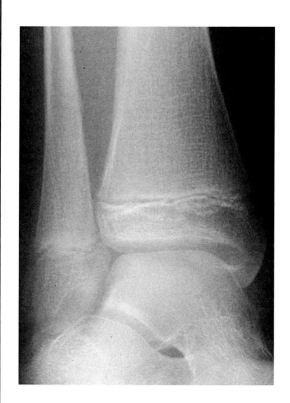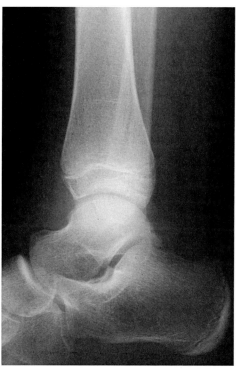

Answer to Case 47

There is an oblique lucent line visualised on the lateral radiograph, which is a fracture. The lucent line is not visible on the anterior-posterior radiograph. It is difficult to assess on these radiographs whether this fracture is of the tibia or fibula, although the lucent line appears to stop at the physeal plate of the tibia (remember that the distal fibular physis should lie at the level of the ankle joint), indicating a fracture of the tibia – a Salter Harris II.

Management of the patient may differ according to whether the fibula or tibia is fractured. If the radiological conclusion of which bone was fractured in this case had not correlated with clinical findings, then oblique radiographs of the ankle would have been helpful. An anterior-posterior radiograph taken 10 days later demonstrates periosteal reaction (callus formation) along the tibial shaft, confirming it was a fracture of the tibia. This radiograph also demonstrates a vertical lucent line in the tibial epiphysis (not visualised previously). This, combined with the fracture demonstrated on the previous lateral, is a triplane fracture (see Case 51).

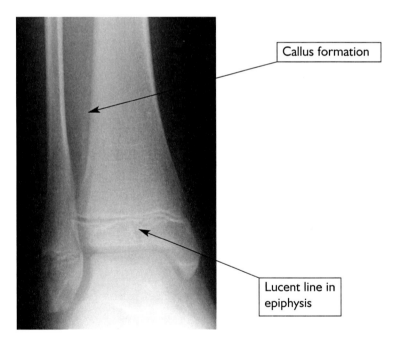

Callus formation

Lucent line in epiphysis

Case 48

Fell whilst playing, plantar flexing foot. Now difficulty weight bearing and generalised pain to ankle.

Write a provisional image evaluation.

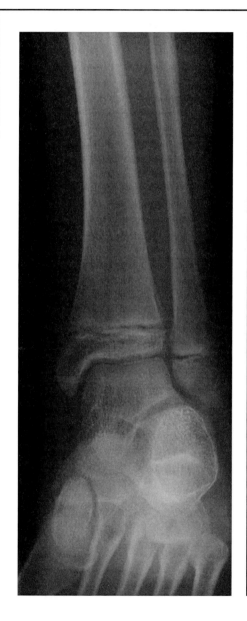 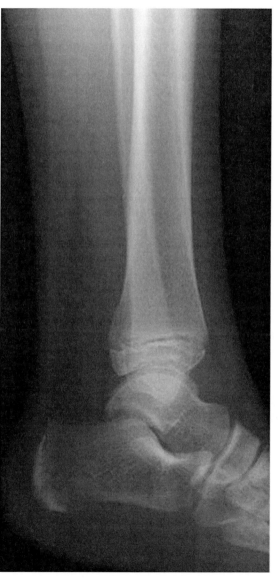

Answer to Case 48

There is a lucent line on the dorsal aspect of distal tibial metaphysis entering the physeal plate. This is a Salter Harris II injury. Injuries involving the physeal plate are just as common in the foot and ankle as other parts of the body.

Sometimes these injuries can be subtle. If suspicious of this injury, an oblique view may be helpful. This injury fits with the mechanism of injury, plantar flexion of the foot. If this was not the case, then a high fibular fracture would need to be ruled out, especially in an adult (the Maissoneuve type fracture), as this would alter patient management.

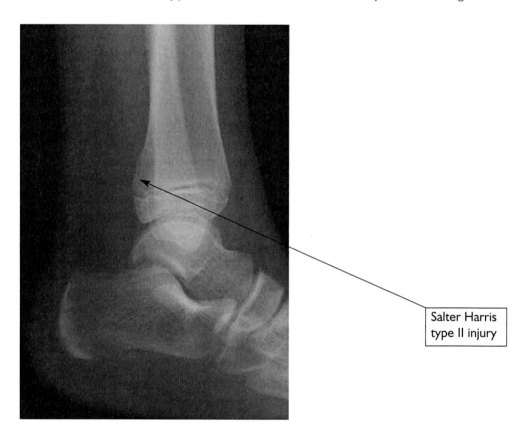

Salter Harris type II injury

Case 49

Patient involved in a rugby tackle, painful ankle ever since. Unsure of mechanism of injury.

Describe the radiographs and classify any injury.

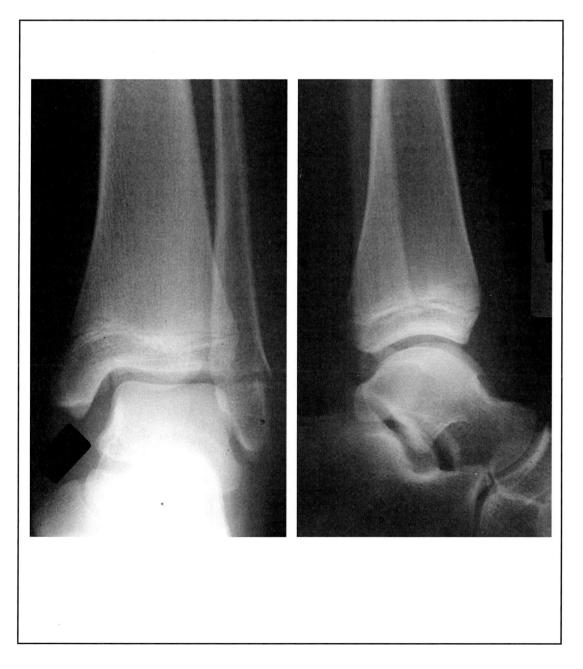

Answer to Case 49

There is a vertical lucent line on the medial aspect of the distal tibia epiphysis, which probably enters the physeal plate. This is a Salter Harris type III injury. There is a widening of the medial joint space. If this was a true mortice view this would be indicative of lateral talar shift, however it is not. Talar shift cannot be assessed on this radiograph (the leg is externally rotated too much). A repeat radiograph with the leg more internally rotated to obtain a true mortice view would be required to assess talar shift.

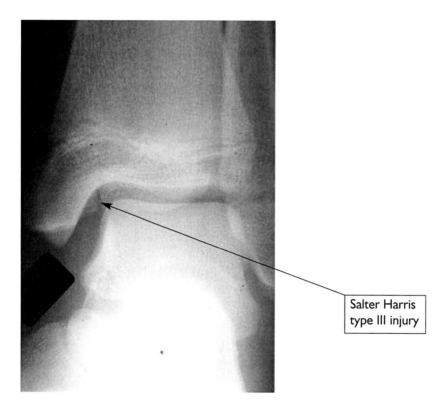

Salter Harris
type III injury

Case 50

Patient twisted ankle, now painful distal fibula.

Describe the radiographs.

Would another view be helpful?

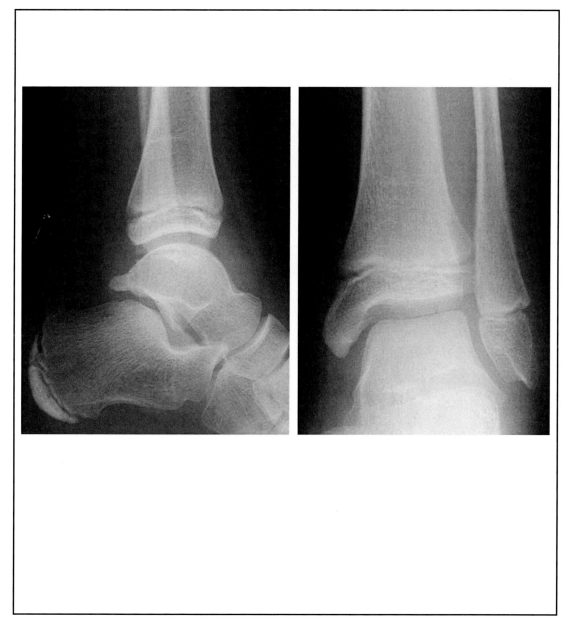

Answer to Case 50

There appears to be a small bony fragment within the posterior ankle joint space, possibly from the fibula. There is also a large joint effusion at the ankle joint. Clinical history suggests injury of the distal fibula. A lateral oblique view of the ankle would demonstrate the distal fibula more clearly. The oblique view demonstrates a Salter Harris II fracture of the distal fibula.

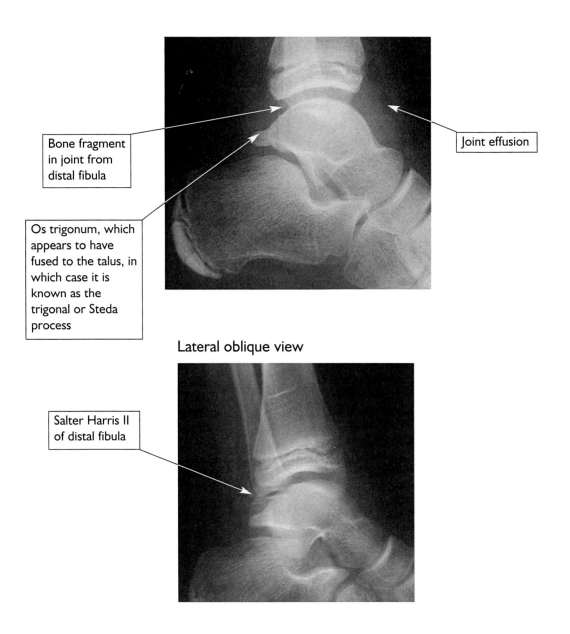

Bone fragment in joint from distal fibula

Joint effusion

Os trigonum, which appears to have fused to the talus, in which case it is known as the trigonal or Steda process

Lateral oblique view

Salter Harris II of distal fibula

Case 51

Patient fell off bicycle, ankle caught in pedals, now painful and swollen.

Describe the radiographs.

What is the name for this type of injury?

Which part of the distal tibial physeal plate is the last to fuse?

Approximately at what age does this occur?

How does this affect trauma to the ankle joint?

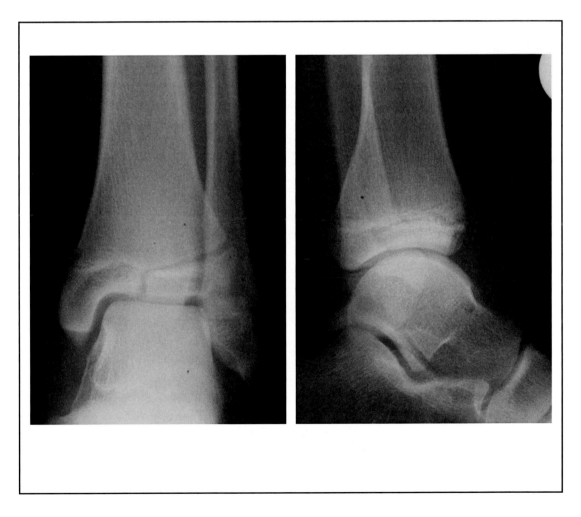

Answer to Case 51

If you review the anterior posterior view there is a vertical lucent line that traverses the epiphysis and there is widening of the lateral tibial physeal plate. If this was classified by Salter Harris it would be a Salter Harris III. At 12.5 years of age the distal tibia physeal plate starts to fuse; the lateral aspect is the last to fuse at about 14 years of age (Figure 7.1); this results in this being a weak area. Remember the physeal plate is weaker than the surrounding ligaments. In an adult following certain mechanisms of injury the ligaments of the distal tibio–fibula syndesmosis will be injured, but in an adolescent with a partially fused distal tibia the same mechanism of injury is more likely to result in a Tillaux fracture (a fracture of the lateral tibial epiphysis).

However if you look at the lateral radiograph then the lucent line can be seen crossing the epiphysis, but there also appears to be another lucent line crossing obliquely the dorsal aspect of the metaphysis. This case demonstrates a triplane fracture – a fracture that crosses three planes, vertically in the epiphysis, transversely in the physeal plate then changes direction again to cross caudally in the metaphysis (as shown in Figure 7.2). They can be divided into two-part injuries or three-part injuries and commonly occur as the distal tibia is fusing (see Figures 7.3, 7.4, 7.5). If you see what looks like a juvenile Tillaux fracture then look very carefully at the dorsal aspect of the distal tibia metaphysis to check that there is not another fracture line and that it is not a juvenile triplane fracture (Figure 7.3). Sometimes computerised axial tomography is useful to demonstrate the extent of injury in triplane fractures. This case is a three-part juvenile triplane fracture.

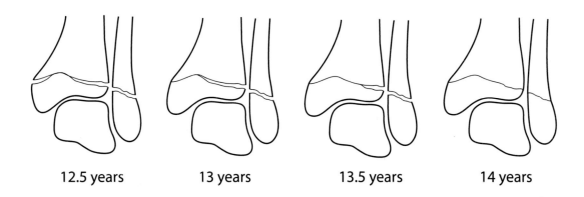

| 12.5 years | 13 years | 13.5 years | 14 years |

Figure 7.1
Pattern of fusion of distal tibia and fibula

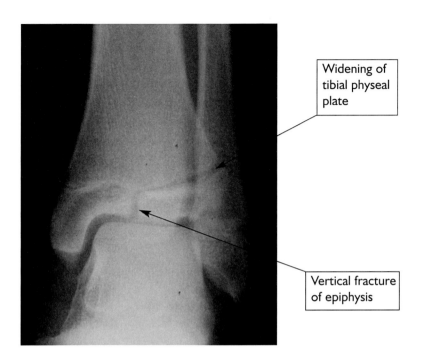

Widening of
tibial physeal
plate

Vertical fracture
of epiphysis

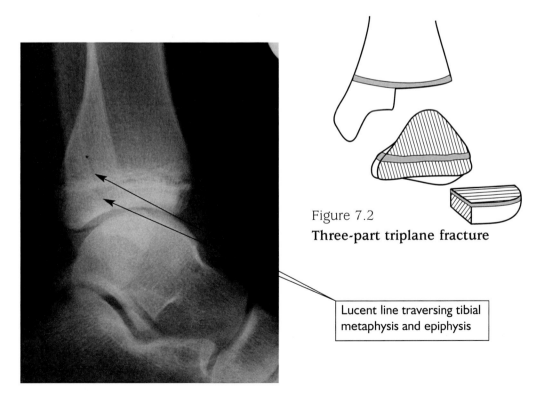

Figure 7.2
Three-part triplane fracture

Lucent line traversing tibial
metaphysis and epiphysis

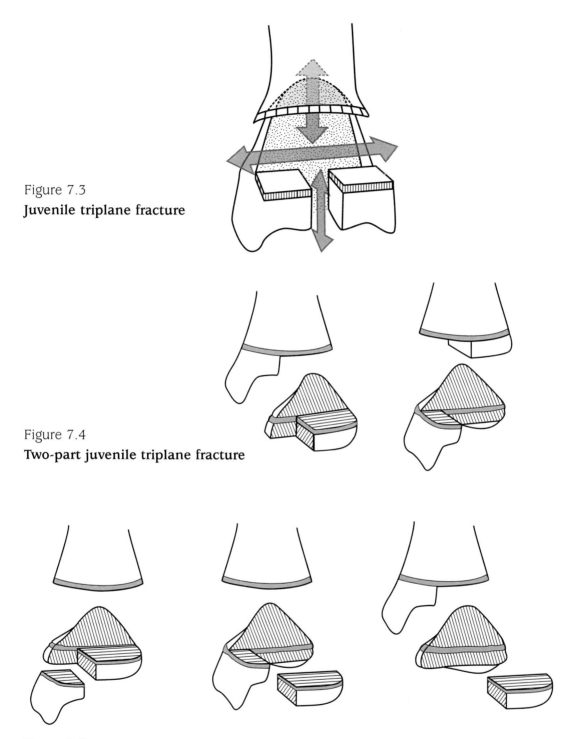

Figure 7.3
Juvenile triplane fracture

Figure 7.4
Two-part juvenile triplane fracture

Figure 7.5
Three-part juvenile triplane fractures

Case 52

Patient fell from climbing frame, injuring ankle.

Describe the radiographs.

What is the name for this type of injury?

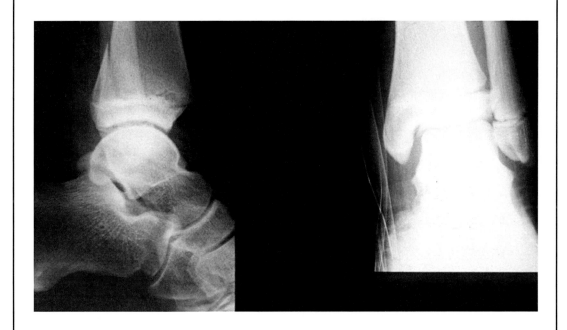

Answer to Case 52

The anterior posterior view demonstrates an oblique fracture through the epiphysis and widening of the physeal plate lateral. This appears to be a Salter Harris type III injury. On reviewing the lateral there is a fracture through the dorsal metaphysis of the tibia, disrupting the physeal plate (the anterior metaphysis and epiphysis of the tibia are no longer in alignment). This appears to be a Salter Harris type II injury. To conclude, this case demonstrates a juvenile triplane fracture (two-part), often a triplane fracture appears as a Salter Harris III on the anterior posterior view, but a Salter Harris II on the lateral view (see Case 51).

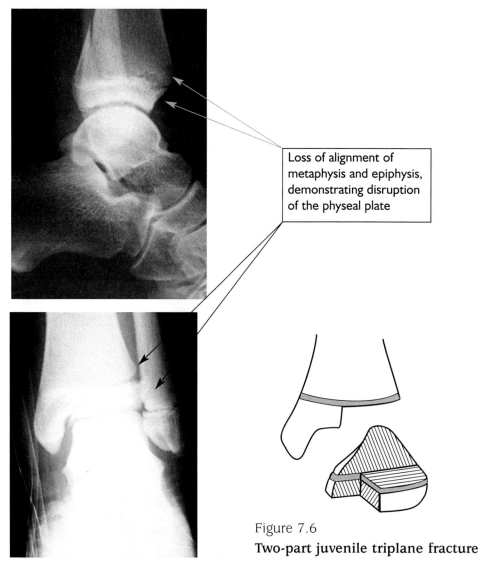

Loss of alignment of metaphysis and epiphysis, demonstrating disruption of the physeal plate

Figure 7.6
Two-part juvenile triplane fracture

Case 53

Patient fell, hit medial malleolus on metal bar, now painful.

Describe the radiographs.

Is there a fracture?

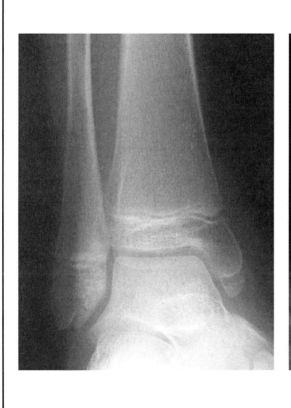 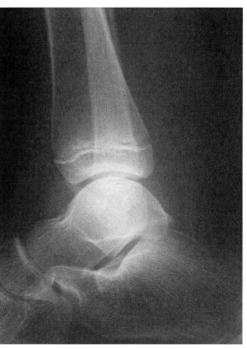

Answer to Case 53

There is a fracture of the medial malleolus. Remember the medial malleolus is made of two parts, called colliculi. The anterior colliculus is long and pointed, the posterior colliculus is short and fat. This is what gives the appearance of a sclerotic line over the medial malleolus, and should not be mistaken as a fracture. In this case there is a step in the cortex and a lucent line distal to the sclerotic line (of the posterior colliculus); hence there is a fracture of the anterior colliculus of the medial malleolus.

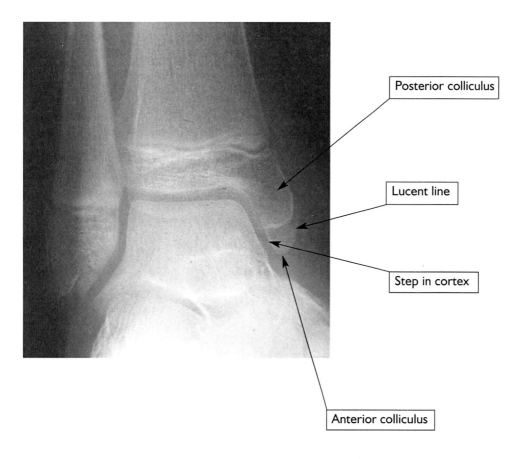

Posterior colliculus

Lucent line

Step in cortex

Anterior colliculus

Case 54

Patient fell down step, inverting ankle, now pain at base of fifth metatarsal.

Describe the radiographs.

Which tendon attaches to the base of the fifth metatarsal?

This tendon lies in close proximity to what other ligament?

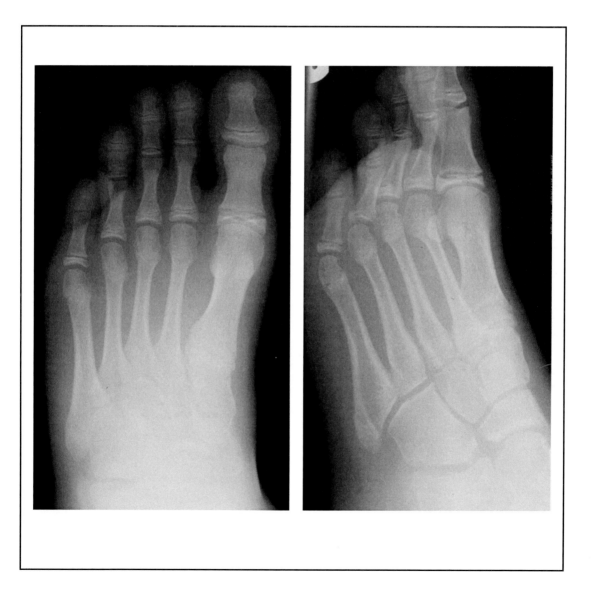

Answer to Case 54

There is a transverse fracture of the base of the fifth metatarsal. The tendon of the peroneus brevis attaches to the base of the fifth metatarsal, and lies in close proximity to the lateral collateral ligament. Inversion of the ankle may stress the lateral collateral ligament resulting in a tear of the ligament or an avulsion fracture of the lateral malleolus, or excessive stress on the peroneus brevis tendon resulting in an avulsion of the base of the fifth metatarsal. Although the clinician when referring for ankle radiography will assess whether there is any bone tenderness to the fifth metatarsal, it is useful in a trauma setting to include the base of the fifth metatarsal on all lateral ankle radiographs to prevent an injury being missed.

With adolescents there is the additional complication of the apophysis at the base of the fifth metatarsal. Apophyses differ from epiphyses in that they do not contribute to longitudinal growth of the bone and are not within a joint. The apophysis at the base of the fifth metatarsal has a vertical orientation, whereas avulsion fractures have a transverse orientation. (Remember the ligament attaches to the inferior border of the base of the fifth metatarsal. Inversion results in a pull inferiorly from the ligaments, resulting in a transverse fracture.)

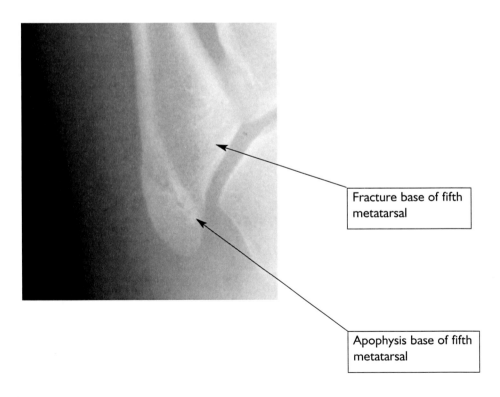

Fracture base of fifth metatarsal

Apophysis base of fifth metatarsal

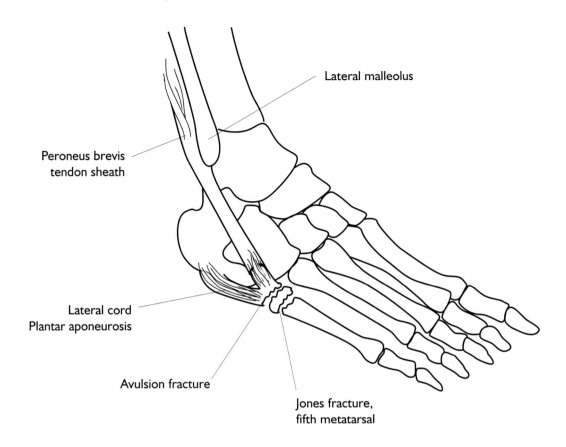

Figure 7.7
Fractures of the base of the fifth metatarsal

Figure 7.7 shows fractures of the base of the fifth metatarsal. These are:
- an avulsion fracture of the base of the fifth metatarsal – occurs secondary to an acute inversion injury.
- a fracture at the junction of the metaphysis and diaphysis of the fifth metatarsal – a stress fracture secondary to overuse.
- a Jones fracture – an acute injury of the fifth metatarsal occurring more distally (2–4 cm distal to the base of the fifth metatarsal).

Jones fractures have a high rate of non-union. Therefore it is important to distinguish between avulsion fractures (which are largely treated conservatively) and Jones fractures which require more formal follow-up and aggressive treatment.

175

Case 55

Patient fell inverting ankle, soft tissue swelling and pain to fifth metatarsal.

Is there a fracture?

Is there an apophysis?

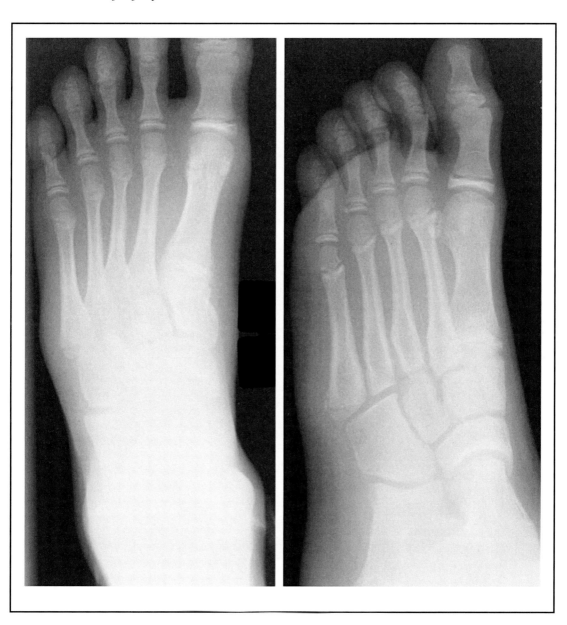

Answer to Case 55

There is a transverse avulsion type fracture of the base of the fifth metatarsal. The apophysis of the base of the fifth metatarsal is also visible (vertically orientated – see Case 54).

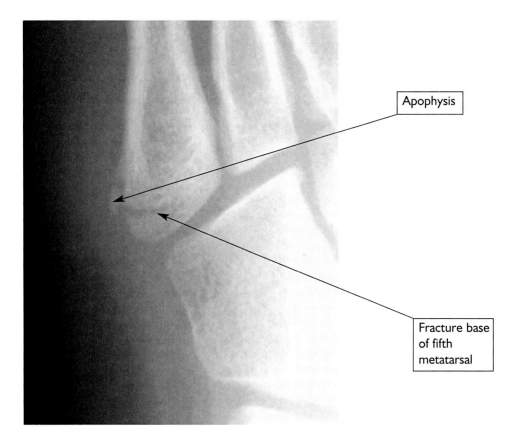

Apophysis

Fracture base of fifth metatarsal

Case 56

Patient stubbed toes, now painful metatarsal heads.

Describe the radiographs.

Is there a fracture?

Are there any normal variants?

Is trauma a common indication for toe radiographs?

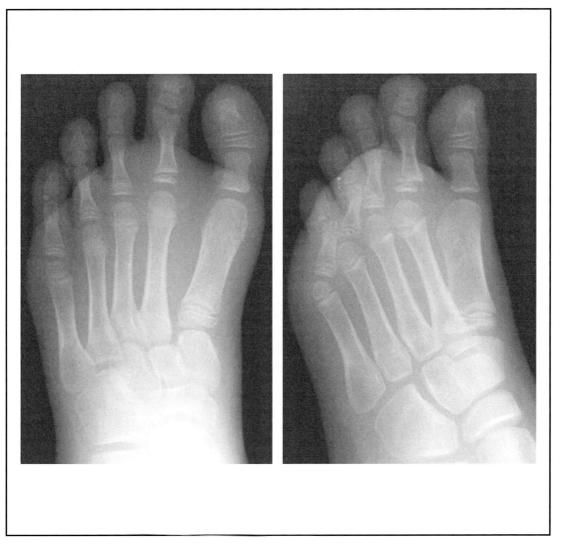

Answer to Case 56

There is a fracture demonstrated on these radiographs. It is a Salter Harris II of the proximal phalanx of the second toe. There are several normal variants demonstrated on this radiograph. Firstly the second toe does not have a middle phalanx. The proximal phalanx of the second toe appears longer than normal, almost as though the proximal phalanx and middle phalanx had fused together (symphalangia). To have no middle phalanx on the second toe is a common normal variant.

A careful look at the hallux reveals that the proximal phalanx is shorter than normal – it does not have an epiphysis, hence no growth, resulting in a shorter proximal phalanx. Also there is a small triangular middle phalanx on the lateral aspect of the fifth (little) toe.

Radiographs should not be taken to demonstrate fractures of the toes as this does not alter management of the patient (see *Making Best Use of a Department of Clinical Radiologists*: Royal College of Radiologists, 2003). However radiographs of the toes may be taken for suspected dislocation, or as in this case when the clinician was querying fracture of the metatarsals (as the results of these radiographs will alter patient management).

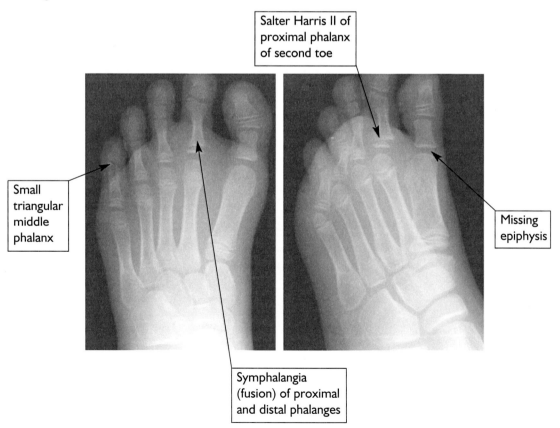

Salter Harris II of proximal phalanx of second toe

Small triangular middle phalanx

Missing epiphysis

Symphalangia (fusion) of proximal and distal phalanges

Case 57

Patient fell twisting foot, painful metatarsal area.

Name the injury. Name the incidental finding.

Comment on some of the causes of the named incidental finding.

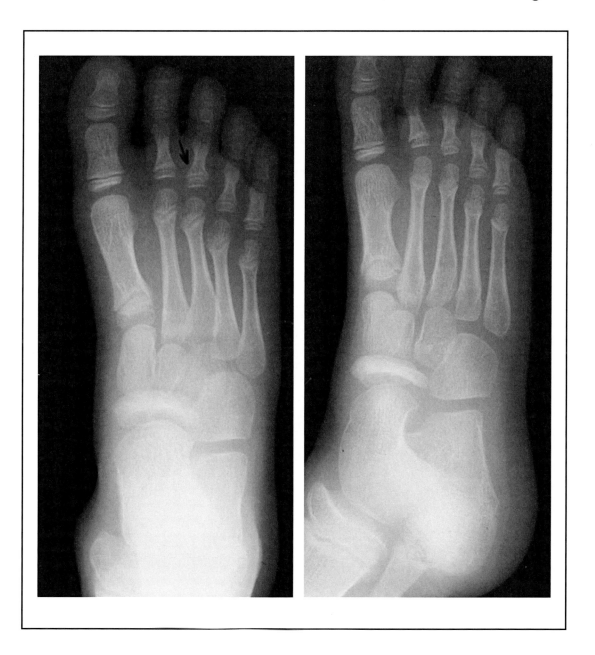

Answer to Case 57

There is a Salter Harris type II fracture of the proximal phalanx of the third toe. The incidental finding is a dense fragmented navicular. This can be a normal variant of ossification that is a self-limited process, which proceeds to normal ossification. But when associated with pain and when a normal navicular has been demonstrated on previous radiographs then it is likely to be Kohler's disease (avascular necrosis of the navicular). Kohler's disease can be idiopathic, or caused by trauma. It may be a result of stress-related compression of the navicular bone at a critical phase of growth. Often seen in boys aged 4 to 10 years of age, presenting with foot pain and limp.

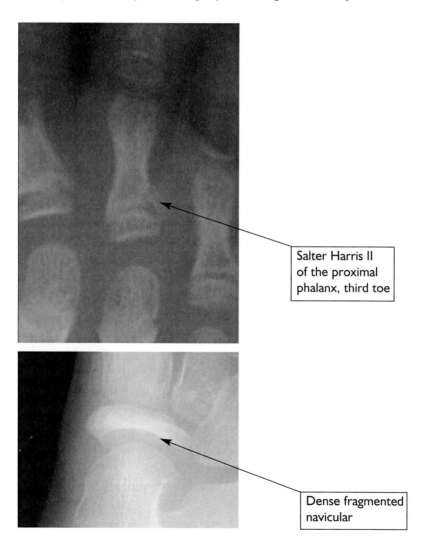

Salter Harris II of the proximal phalanx, third toe

Dense fragmented navicular

Case 58

Patient's sibling hit him with a toy car, metatarsal area, now bruising, pain and non-weight bearing.

Describe the radiographs.

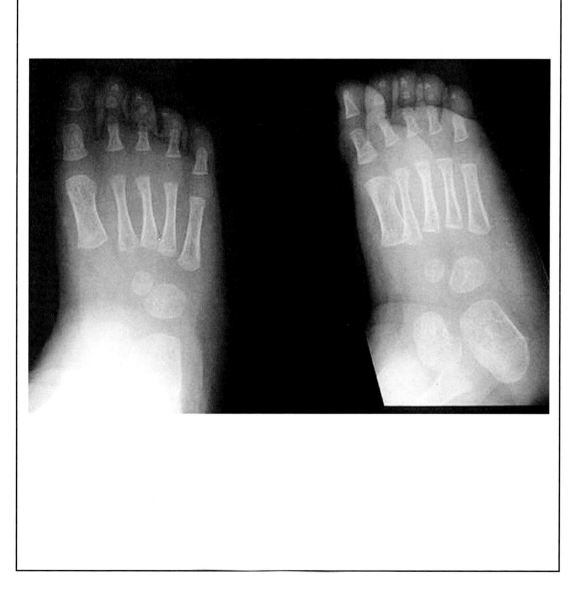

Answer to Case 58

There are buckle fractures of the distal third, medial aspect of third and fourth metatarsals. This coincided with the area of impact and bruising.

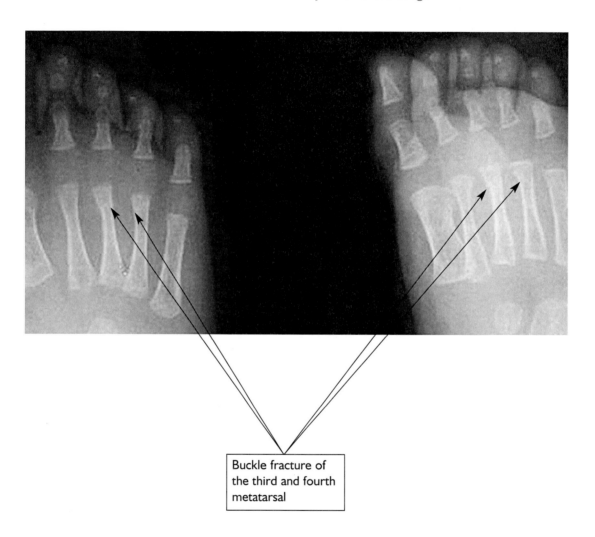

Buckle fracture of
the third and fourth
metatarsal

Case 59

Patient stubbed hallux on steps then proceeded to fall down the steps. Pain in hallux, with limited weight bearing.

Is there an injury? If so name it.

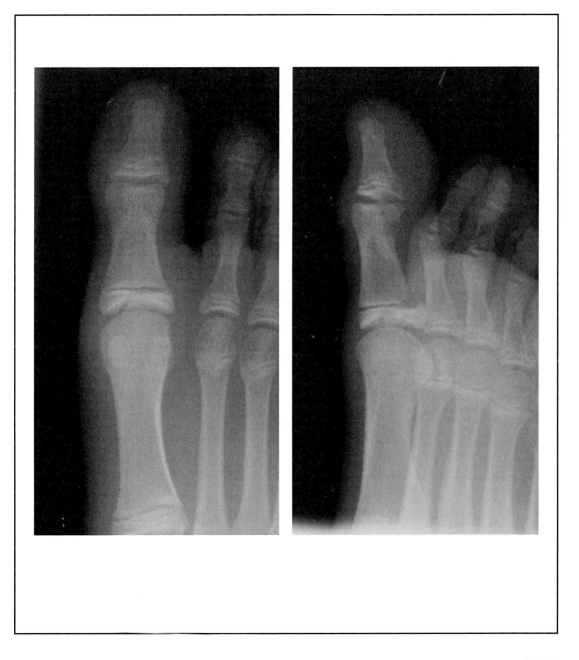

Answer to Case 59

There is an oblique lucent line in the epiphysis of the hallux, with a widening of the physeal plate dorsally. This is a Salter Harris type III injury. Be careful, though, that a bifid epiphysis of the base of the proximal phalanx is not mistaken for a Salter Harris type III injury. With a bifid epiphysis there would be no disruption of the physeal plate as demonstrated in this case.

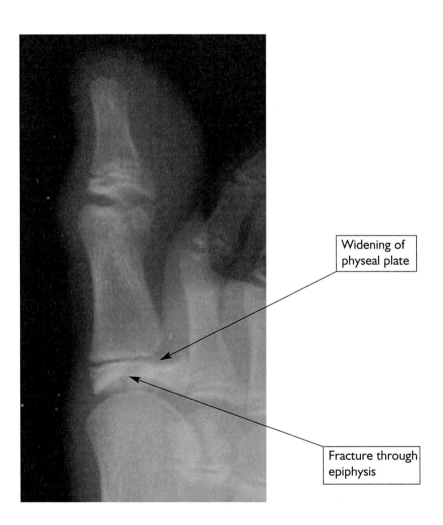

Widening of physeal plate

Fracture through epiphysis

Case 60

Patient fell, twisting ankle. Now pain distal fibula and non-weight bearing.

Is there an injury?

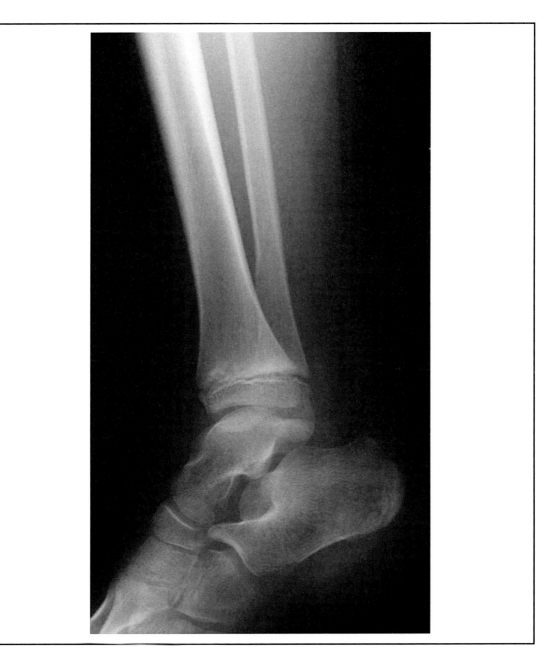

Answer to Case 60

Unfortunately no antero-posterior view is available. An overturned lateral radiograph was taken to better demonstrate the distal fibula, as the pain/injury was associated with this area. A buckle type fracture is demonstrated at the distal fibula.

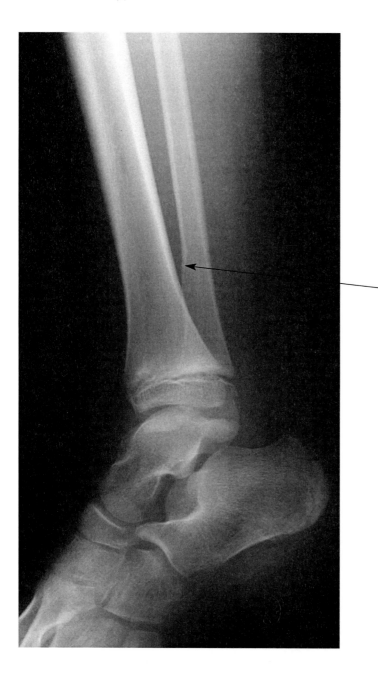

Buckle of
distal fibula

Case 61

Patient jumped off a shed roof, bony tender calcaneum.

Write a provisional image evaluation.

If there is a fracture, can it be classified using the Salter Harris classification?

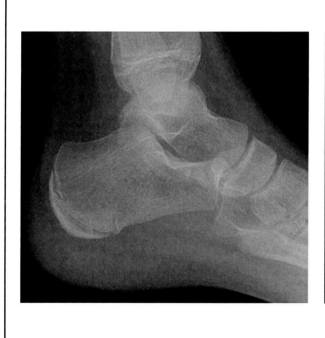
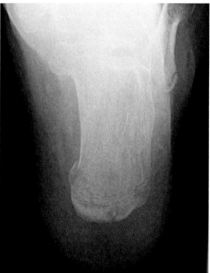

Answer to Case 61

There is an oblique fracture involving the medial aspect of the metaphysis and apophysis of the calcaneum. As the fracture does not involve the epiphysis, it cannot be classified using the Salter Harris classification system. Refer back to Chapter 2 if you have forgotten the difference between an epiphysis and an apophysis.

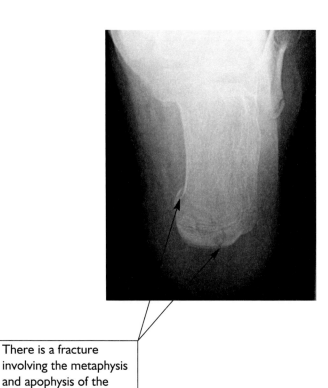

There is a fracture involving the metaphysis and apophysis of the calcaneum

Case 62

Patient fell from bicycle, general bony tenderness over foot.

Write a provisional image evaluation.

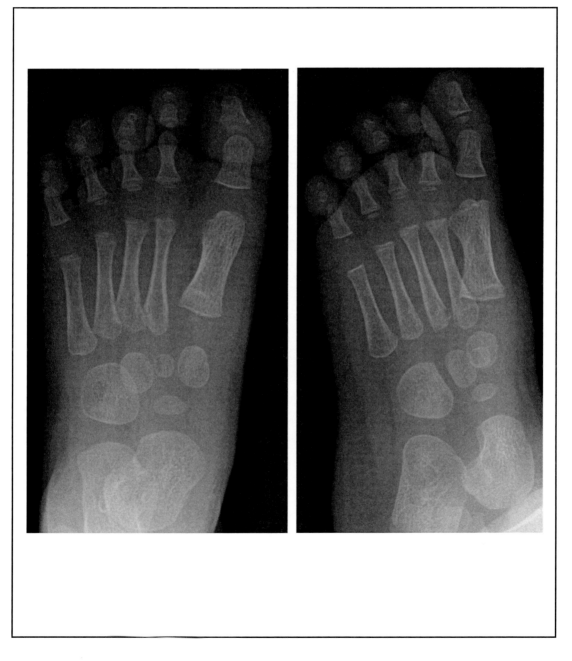

Answer to Case 62

In this case there is no bony injury. This is sometimes the most difficult report to obtain, especially in paediatrics, as one is often frightened of missing something subtle. The best strategy is to look at lots of normal paediatric images, including those with 'normal variants'. This will make it easier to recognise an abnormal image, whether due to trauma or pathology.

Case 63

Patient fell from bicycle, injuring ankle.

Write a provisional image evaluation.

If there is an injury, can it be classified using the Salter Harris classification system?

After you have come to your conclusions, is there another area that you should review to ensure that a significant injury is not missed?

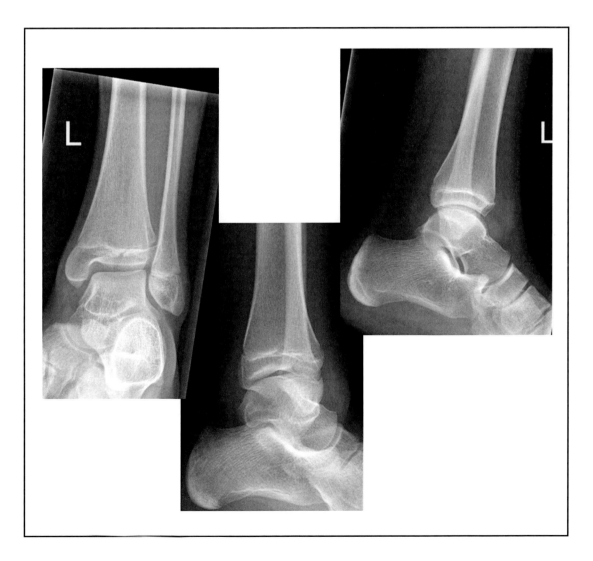

Answer to Case 63

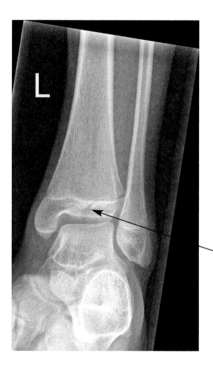

Lucent line at tibial epiphysis, with widening of tibial physis laterally, a Salter Harris type III injury

There is a lucent line at the tibial epiphysis, with widening of tibial physis laterally; this is a Salter Harris type III injury. With this injury, one should review carefully whether there is a second fracture line of the posterior tibial metaphysis. This would be a juvenile triplane injury and would significantly alter patient management, as it is a serious injury requiring CT and internal fixation. In this case no further fractures were demonstrated. The oblique was helpful in assessing for further fractures.

Case 64

Patient jumped from garden wall, injuring ankle. There is no bony tenderness to the calcaneum.

Write a provisional image evaluation.

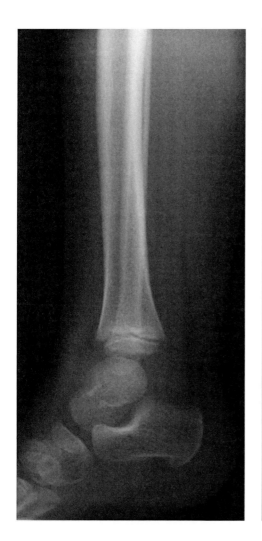
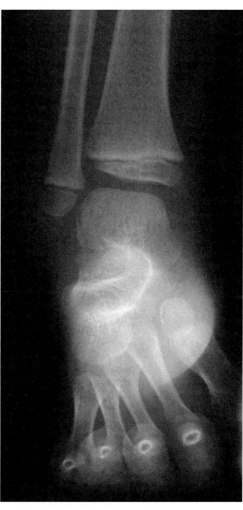

Answer to Case 64

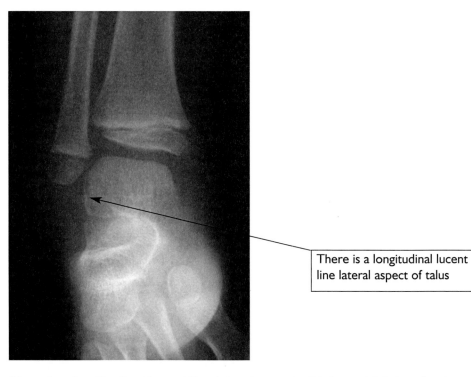

There is a longitudinal lucent line lateral aspect of talus

There is a longitudinal lucent line lateral aspect of talus, which is a fracture. Often, when jumping from a height, the calcaneum is injured, as it is the initial point of impact. In this case, the mechanism of force has been transferred through the calcaneum up to the talus, resulting in a longitudinal fracture of the lateral aspect of the talus.

Case 65

Fell whilst playing, plantar flexing foot, now difficulty weight bearing and generalised pain to ankle.

Write a provisional image evaluation.

Would other views be helpful?

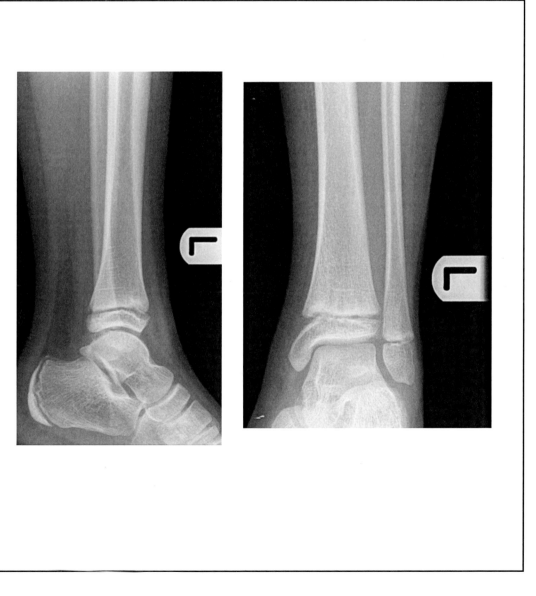

Answer to Case 65

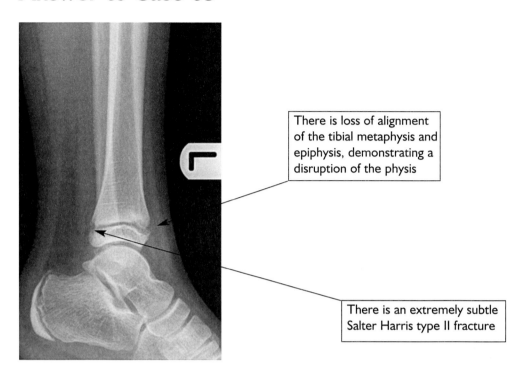

There is loss of alignment of the tibial metaphysis and epiphysis, demonstrating a disruption of the physis

There is an extremely subtle Salter Harris type II fracture

There is an extremely subtle un-displaced Salter Harris type II fracture of the dorsal aspect of the distal tibia, which could easily be missed if this area was not reviewed carefully.

Oblique views may have been helpful if the reporter was doubtful about the injury. But there are other clues to the injury: there is loss of alignment of the tibial metaphysis and epiphysis, demonstrating a definite disruption of the physis.

The patient was x-rayed again 10 days later. Periosteal reaction is now demonstrated along the tibia, confirming a healing fracture. The lateral image differs slightly from the original in position, and there now appears to be a fracture fragment from the anterior metaphysis of the distal tibia as well as the posterior.

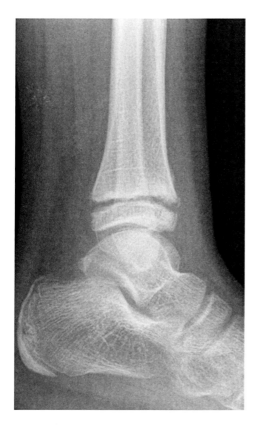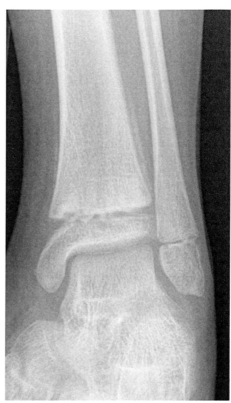

8.

Knee, tibia and fibula trauma

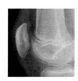

Case 66

Patient fell from climbing frame injuring knee, now painful, limited weight bearing.

Describe the radiograph?

Is there an injury?

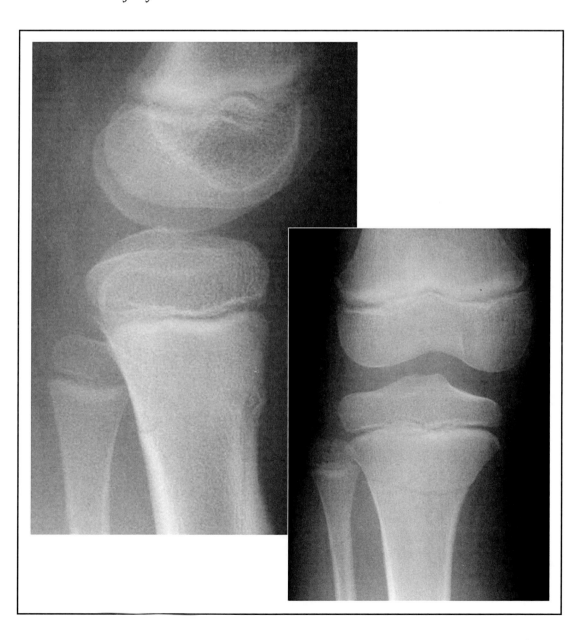

Answer to Case 66

The lateral view demonstrates a buckle of the proximal tibia; if you look carefully there is a lucent line. The lateral view also demonstrates a faint lucent line traversing the proximal fibula. The anterior posterior view clearly demonstrates the fracture of the proximal tibia – it is a greenstick fracture. The anteroposterior view also demonstrates the lucent line again on the proximal fibula. Hence, as it is demonstrated on both views, it is a definite fracture.

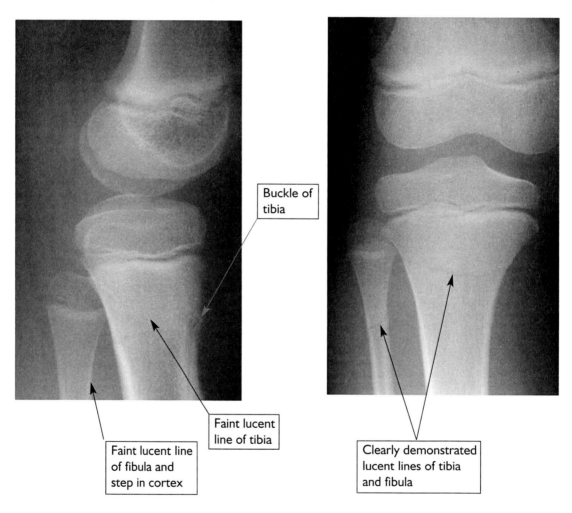

Buckle of tibia

Faint lucent line of tibia

Faint lucent line of fibula and step in cortex

Clearly demonstrated lucent lines of tibia and fibula

Epiphyseal injuries may also occur in the knee, but are relatively rare, Salter Harris II being the most common (70 per cent of physeal injuries of the knee).

The knee, however, is the most common site for a Salter Harris type V injury. They are usually seen in the proximal tibia and are associated with tibial shaft fractures.

Case 67

Patient presented to accident and emergency after limping for 2 days, no definite history of trauma. On clinical examination there is bony tenderness over tibia.

Describe the radiograph.

Is there an injury? If so, what is the common mechanism of injury?

In what age group does this normally occur?

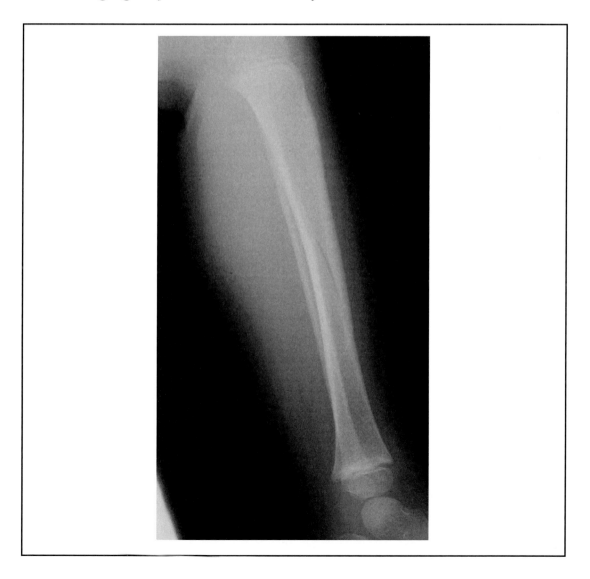

Answer to Case 67

There is an undisplaced fracture of the mid-shaft of the tibia. Unfortunately the anterior posterior view is no longer available, but the fracture was not demonstrated on that radiograph. This is commonly called a toddler's fracture; often they are undisplaced and only visible on one radiographic view. Commonly the patient presents to accident and emergency with an acute onset of a limp, without a clear history of trauma. Normally these injuries occur at about 2 years of age; when the child is learning to walk, they fall over, keeping their leg straight, which puts torsion on the calf and resulting in an undisplaced fracture. Recent thinking suggests that for a fracture to be viewed radiographically it must be displaced, so it is perhaps more accurate to describe a fracture such as this as minimally displaced.

In a child of this age, if no fracture is demonstrated on either view, a repeat radiograph in 7 to 10 days may reveal a healing response rendering the fracture detectable.

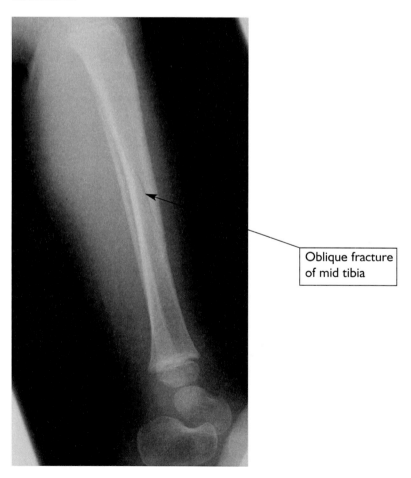

Oblique fracture of mid tibia

Case 68

Patient fell from bicycle, now painful knee, unable to weight bear.

Describe the radiographs.

Comment on the type of lateral knee view performed in a trauma situation.

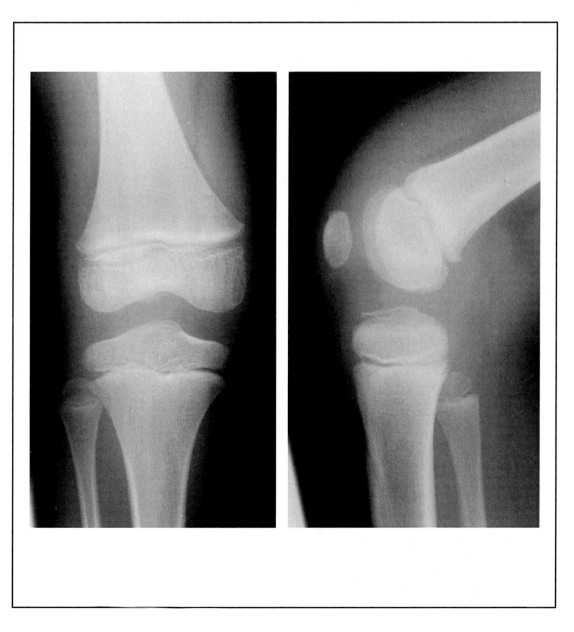

Answer to Case 68

There is an avulsion of the anterior tibial spine at the insertion of the anterior cruciate ligament. This is a common injury in children and adolescents, and occurs at the origin of the anterior cruciate ligament. Over 50 per cent of these injuries are caused by falls from a bicycle, the normal mechanism of injury being hyperextension.

In the trauma situation a horizontal beam knee radiograph should always be taken. This allows assessment of joint effusion (expansion of the suprapatellar bursa to more than 5 mm), and whether a lipohaemoarthrosis is present or not (Figure 8.1). A lipohaemoarthrosis is demonstrated radiographically by a fat fluid level at the supra-patella bursa. A lipohaemoarthrosis is always indicative of fracture, even if no fracture line is demonstrated radiographically, as the only way fat can be in the soft tissue is if it has escaped from the bone marrow following fracture.

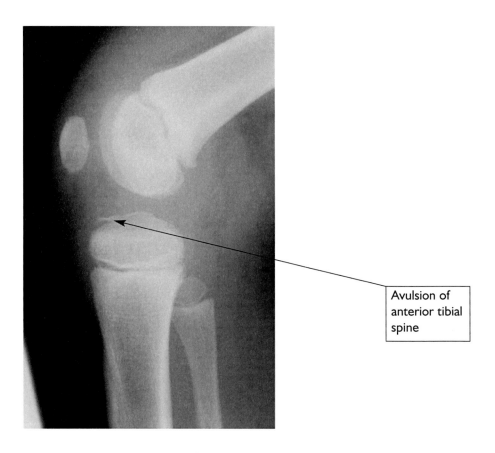

Avulsion of anterior tibial spine

Horizontal beam lateral radiograph of normal knee

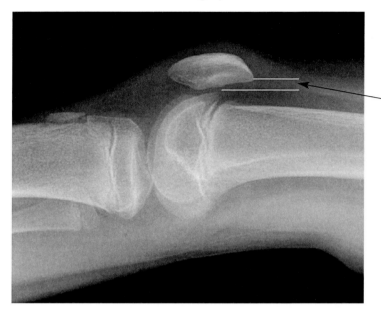

Normal width of suprapatella bursa – hence no joint effusion

Horizontal beam lateral radiograph demonstrating a joint effusion

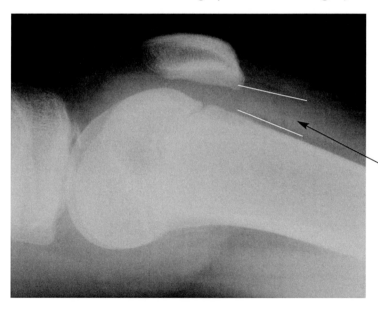

Widened suprapatella bursa indicative of a joint effusion

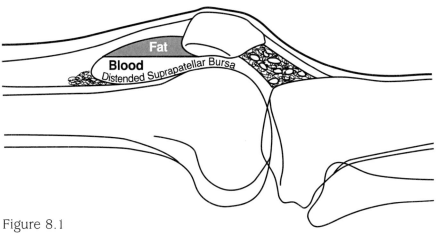

Figure 8.1

Lipohaemoarthrosis: a horizontal beam lateral radiograph

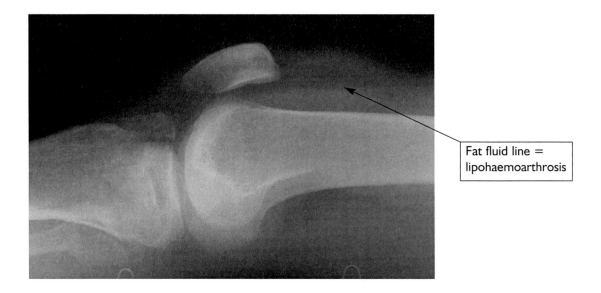

Fat fluid line =
lipohaemoarthrosis

Case 69

Patient fell from bicycle, now non-weight bearing, unable to straighten knee.

Describe the radiographs.

Which ligament is involved?

Why is the intercondylar notch seen on the anterior posterior radiograph?

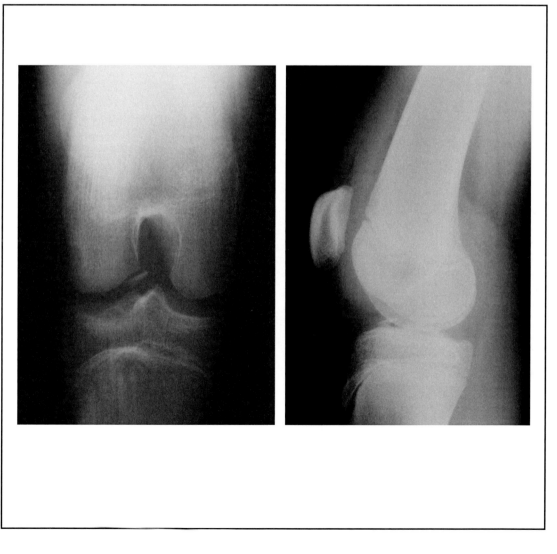

Answer to Case 69

There is an avulsion of the anterior tibial spine, at the insertion of the anterior cruciate ligament (see Case 68). The horizontal beam lateral radiograph demonstrates that the avulsion is from the anterior tibial spine, and also demonstrates a joint effusion. The intercondylar notch is seen on the anterior posterior radiograph because the patient is unable to straighten their knee, thereby producing the so called 'tunnel view' projection.

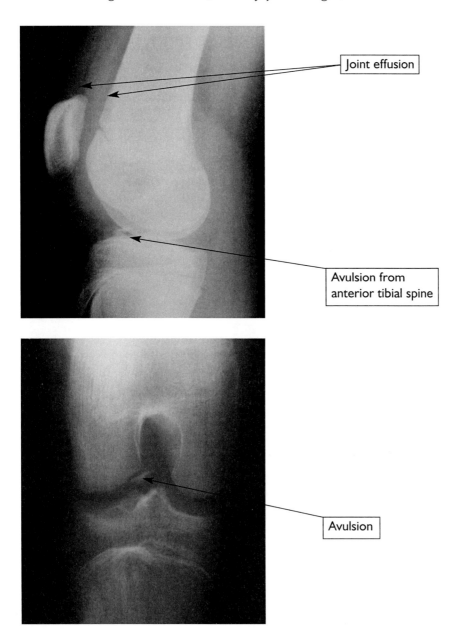

Joint effusion

Avulsion from
anterior tibial spine

Avulsion

Case 70

Patient jumped down several steps, now painful knee, particularly over anterior tibial tubercle.

Describe the radiograph.

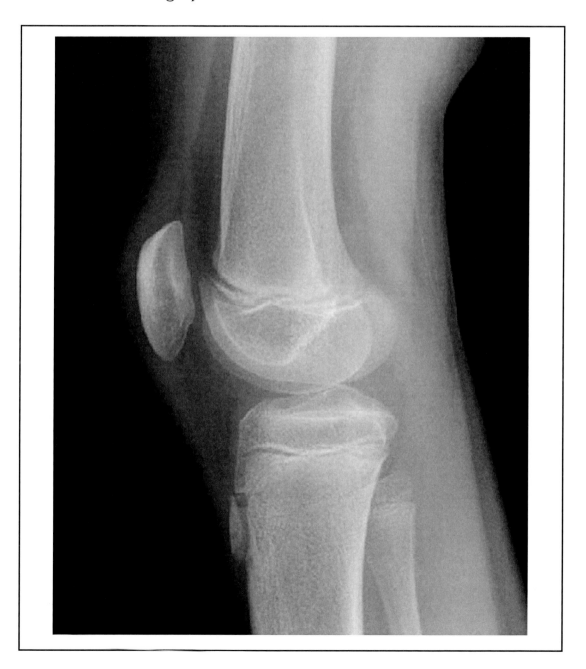

Answer to Case 70

There is no bony injury demonstrated on this one radiograph as the tibial tubercle is frequently fragmented, and should not be mistaken for a fracture. However the tibial tubercle can fracture, and frequently follows a 'jumping' injury. It is a common injury in adolescents. The fracture may involve just the tibial tubercle or extend back into the physeal plate. No joint effusion is demonstrated on the horizontal beam lateral radiograph (although one would not be expected with a tibial spine injury).

Normal tibial apophysis

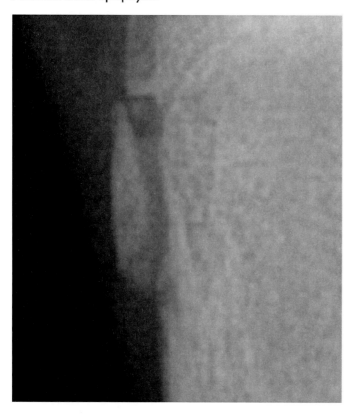

Case 71

Patient jumped down from climbing frame, twisting knee.

Describe the radiograph.

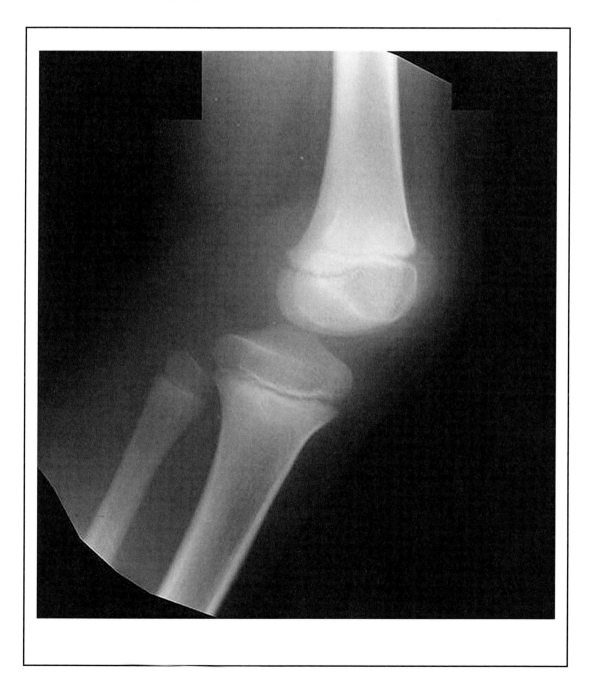

Answer to Case 71

Unfortunately there is no anterior posterior view available. This radiograph demonstrates dislocation of the patella. There is no joint space between the inferior aspect of the patella and superior aspect of the distal femur (the patella appears to lie to one side of the femur instead of in front of it). Patellae normally dislocate laterally, but as there is no anterior posterior view we cannot be sure of this (see Case 73).

Case 72

Adolescent patient fell, twisting knee, now painful to walk

Describe the radiograph.

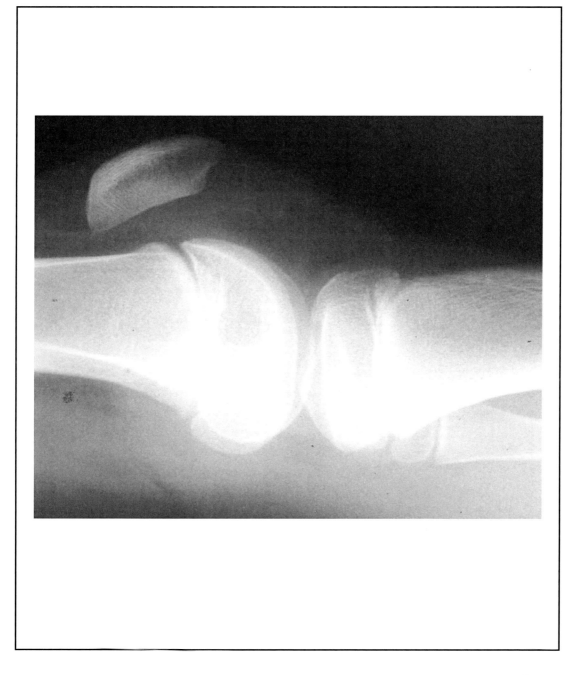

Answer to Case 72

The inferior pole of the patella is raised superiorly; in this area there is a fragment of bone. This is an osteochondral fragment. They commonly occur in adolescents and adults. Mechanism of injury is usually a force directed tangentially to the joint. Common areas for this type of injury are the femoral condyles, talus and capitellum. When just a chondral fragment (i.e. with no bony component) is present, magnetic resonance imaging is required for adequate demonstration.

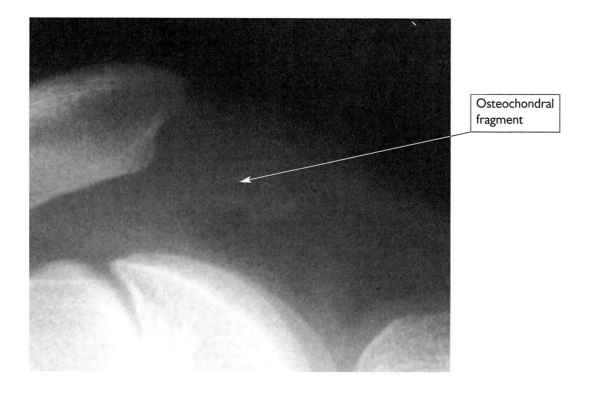

Osteochondral fragment

Case 73

Patient involved in a road traffic incident. Painful knee, arrived in ambulance with a leg splint on.

Can you see an injury without the benefit of a lateral view?

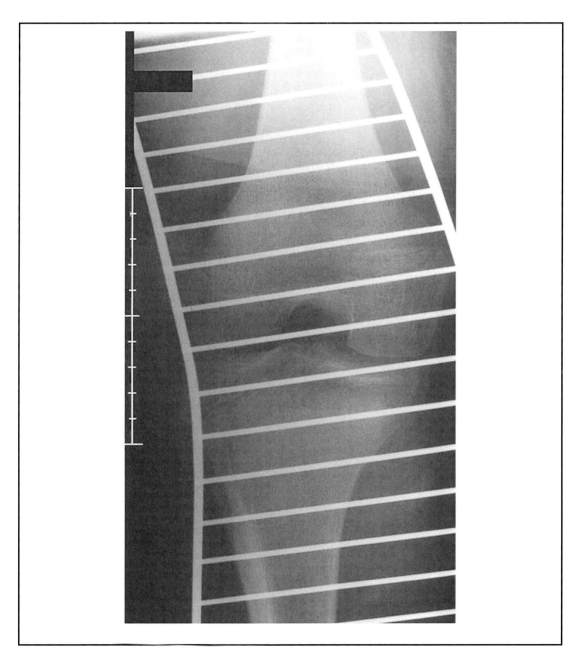

Answer to Case 73

The splint is very distracting and may hide subtle fractures; consequently it should have been removed prior to x-ray. But a careful look reveals the injury; a lateral dislocation of the patella, which is readily demonstrated on the lateral radiograph.

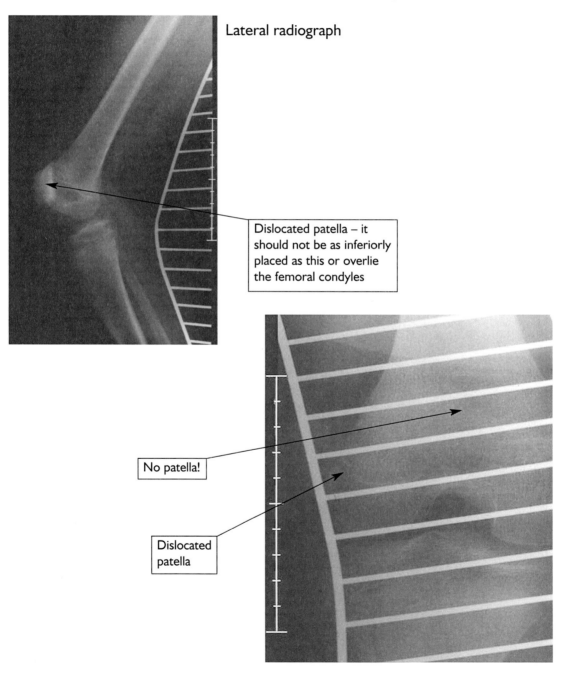

Lateral radiograph

Dislocated patella – it should not be as inferiorly placed as this or overlie the femoral condyles

No patella!

Dislocated patella

Patella dislocation is normally lateral. Patients with patella alta (the patella lies in a higher position relative to the femur than normal), patella tilt and lateral patella displacement are more prone to lateral dislocation or subluxation of the patella. Sometimes the patella as it dislocates can knock off a fragment of bone, which may remain in the joint resulting in reduced movement and locking. Patella alta can be viewed on the lateral knee radiograph (it is elongation of the infrapatella tendon). On the turned lateral view of the knee, with 20 to 30 degrees flexion, the ratio of the infrapatella tendon length (from the inferior pole of the patella to the anterior tubercle) to the length of the patella is 1.0 ±0.2 (Figure 8.2). If this ratio is greater than 1.2, patella alta exists (see Figure 8.3).

This view is normally taken with the knee flexed by 20 degrees. As such, it is not usually performed in A&E if the patella is still obviously dislocated, but is normally requested by an orthopaedic practitioner in a follow-up clinic. However, these days if the patella dislocation has spontaneously reduced, or there is suspicion of remaining subluxed patella, then the skyline view is routinely performed in the A&E department, providing the patient is able to flex their knee. This also allows assessment for associated osteochondral fractures.

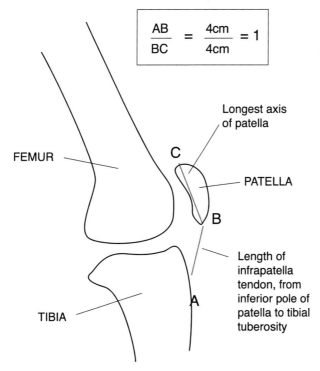

Figure 8.2
Normal infrapatellar tendon:patella ratio

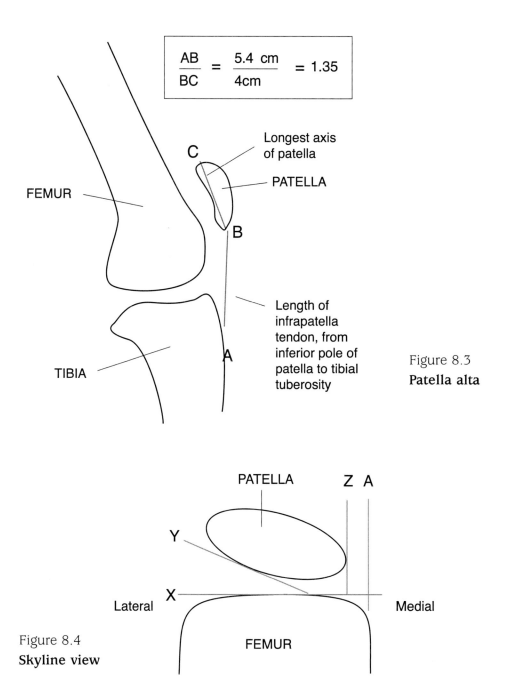

$$\frac{AB}{BC} = \frac{5.4 \text{ cm}}{4 \text{cm}} = 1.35$$

C — Longest axis of patella

PATELLA

FEMUR

B

Length of infrapatella tendon, from inferior pole of patella to tibial tuberosity

TIBIA

A

Figure 8.3
Patella alta

PATELLA   Z A

Y

X
Lateral   Medial

Figure 8.4
Skyline view

FEMUR

X and Y form an angle that normally opens laterally, if it opened medially then there is patella tilt. Line A is perpendicular to line X and at the tip of the medial femoral condyle, line Z is one millimetre lateral to line A and normally intersects the medial patella; if it does not, the patella is laterally displaced and prone to subluxation.

Case 74

Patient fell off skateboard, then fell again as moving away from other skateboarders. Very painful knee, non-weight bearing.

Describe the radiograph.

Would another view be helpful?

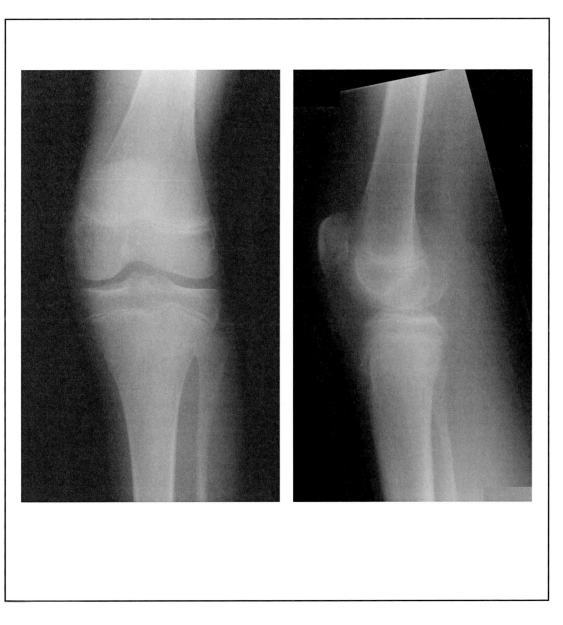

Answer to Case 74

There is a torus fracture of the proximal fibula, and an oblique fracture of the fibula more distally. The lateral aspect of the tibial metaphysis demonstrates an irregularity of the cortex, which is probably a fracture. The lateral knee is not a true lateral and was repeated, clearly demonstrating an avulsion type fracture of the posterior aspect of the tibial metaphysis. A careful look at this area reveals the fracture transversing the whole tibia. It is unusual to get two fractures of the fibula, but this case demonstrates the importance of looking very carefully at the whole radiograph even when one fracture has already been identified.

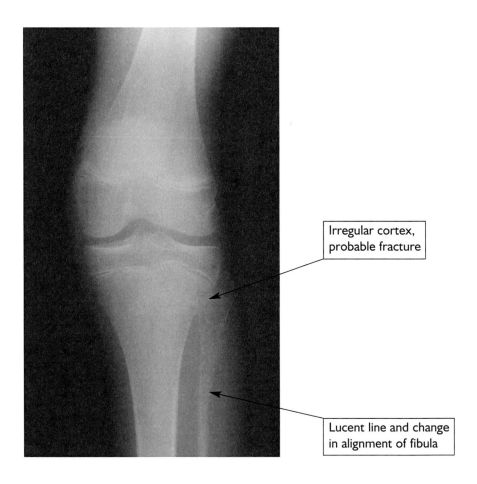

Irregular cortex, probable fracture

Lucent line and change in alignment of fibula

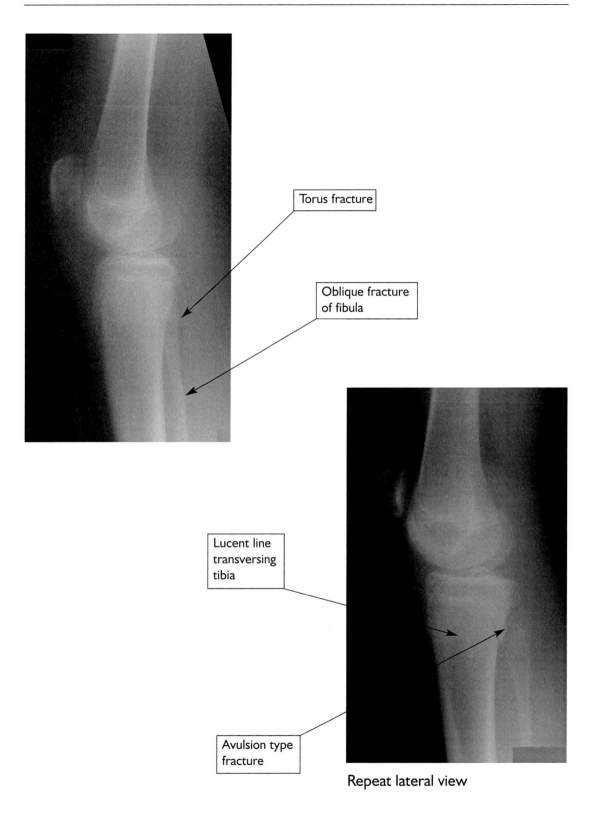

Torus fracture

Oblique fracture of fibula

Lucent line transversing tibia

Avulsion type fracture

Repeat lateral view

225

Case 75

Patient fell whilst skipping, painful tibia and fibula.

Describe the radiographs.

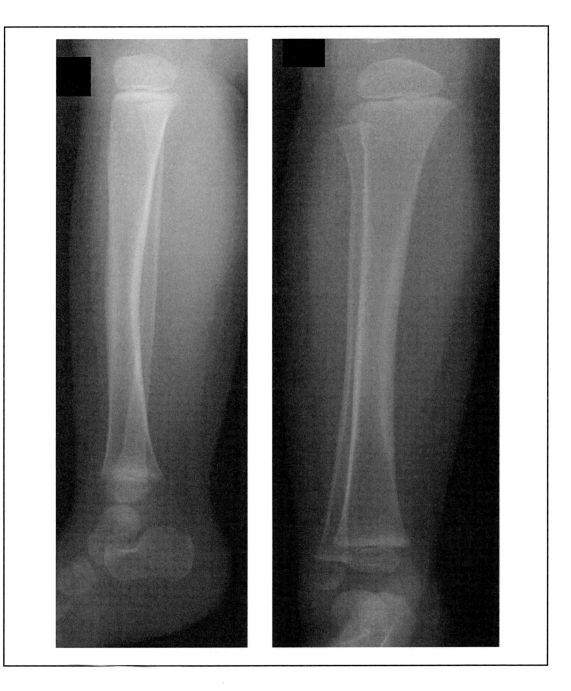

Answer to Case 75

There is a torus fracture of the proximal tibia (lateral aspect) and a buckle type fracture of the fibula at the same level. This demonstrates the importance of looking carefully at the whole length of both bones on tibia and fibula radiographs, particularly close to both joints (remember the tibia and fibula form a ring-like structure; if you see one injury, look for another). Review the proximal tibia again and it reveals a break in the cortex medial aspect. Hence this is a 'lead pipe' type fracture (see Chapter 2).

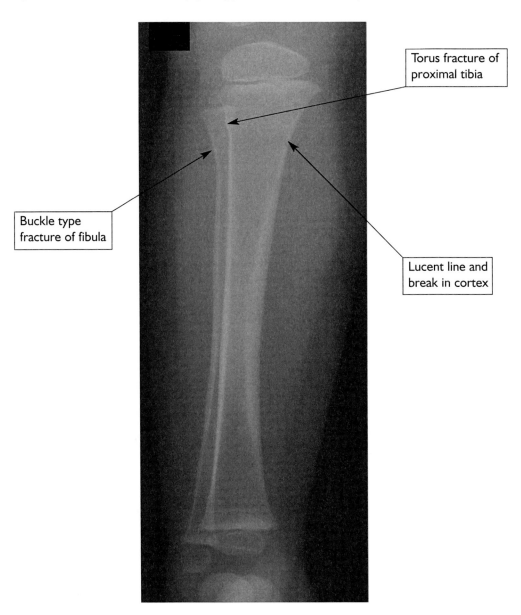

Torus fracture of proximal tibia

Buckle type fracture of fibula

Lucent line and break in cortex

This case demonstrates clearly the difference between a torus fracture and a buckle fracture, although often the terms are used interchangeably to describe the same thing. Buckle fractures appear radiographically as a sharp change in angulation of the cortex, and appear on only one view, while a torus fracture is often demonstrated on more than one view and is rounded in appearance. Think of the moulded profiles of old fashioned skirting boards or the bases of Greek columns – torus fractures look like this (see Figure 8.5). See also cases 15 and 19.

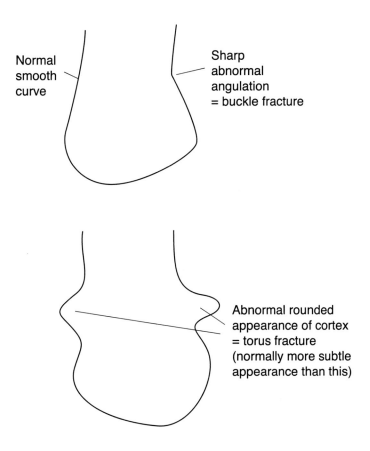

Normal smooth curve

Sharp abnormal angulation = buckle fracture

Abnormal rounded appearance of cortex = torus fracture (normally more subtle appearance than this)

Figure 8.5
Buckle and torus fractures

9.

Pelvis and hip trauma

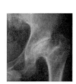

Case 76

Adolescent patient fell whilst running in games, now painful left hip.

Is there an injury demonstrated on this pelvic radiograph? (View the pelvis before looking at the lateral hip radiograph on the next page.)

In what age group does this injury take place?

Discuss some of the clues found on anterior posterior radiographs to this injury.

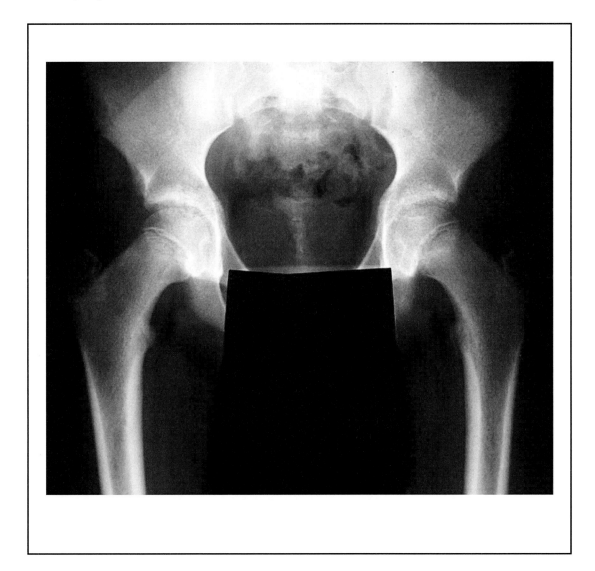

Answer to Case 76

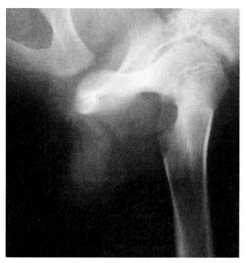

The radiographs demonstrate a slipped femoral epiphysis on the left side. The injury is demonstrated on the pelvis radiograph, and confirmed on the lateral. A lateral radiograph is not always required to confirm this injury – however it is always required to exclude slipped capital femoral epiphysis if this is suspected and it is the patient's first presentation. This is because subtle slips may be missed on the anterior posterior view. Slipped capital femoral epiphysis is a disorder of adolescence – the femoral head appears to slip posteriorly and inferiorly. In fact the femoral head does not move at all; it remains in joint with normal congruity with the acetabulum. What moves is the femoral shaft. Boys are more often affected than girls, particularly overweight, 'Pickwickian' types. This injury tends to occur during the years of rapid growth (10 to 16 years of age), during which the femoral neck changes from valgus to varus; this puts further stress on a growth plate already weakened by rapid growth, hence minor trauma may result in slipped femoral epiphysis. Some studies suggest that an imbalance between growth hormones and sex hormones weakens the physeal plate, rendering it more vulnerable to the shearing forces of weight bearing and injury.

On the anterior posterior radiograph the physeal plate appears wider, with less distinct margins, the epiphysis appears shorter and there is loss of the triangular sign of Capener (a very subtle sign). A line drawn along the lateral femoral neck normally intersects a small amount of the femoral epiphysis (the lateral sixth of the femoral epiphysis) but when the epiphysis has slipped it does not. Remember the pelvis demonstrates both hips so you can compare one side to the other. Disuse osteoporosis of the femoral neck and head may also be demonstrated, on the affected side in chronic cases or acutely on chronic cases (the frog lateral, or horizontal beam lateral radiograph, normally confirms the diagnosis). Figure 9.1 demonstrates the clues to injury on the anterior posterior radiograph, normal being to the left, abnormal to the right.

This case shows the patient with gonad shielding. Normally (in our hospital) at first presentation gonad shielding is not used on anterior posterior or lateral radiographs for females; with males it depends on the area of interest, and is not used in trauma. At second presentation gonad shielding should be used on both sexes on both anterior posterior and lateral views.

234

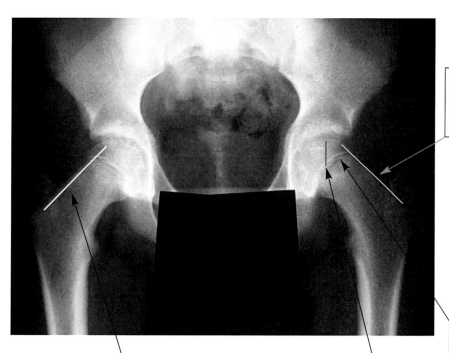

Line along femoral neck no longer intersects epiphysis

Wider indistinct physeal plate

Normal hip – line along femoral neck intersects epiphysis

Loss of height of the epiphysis

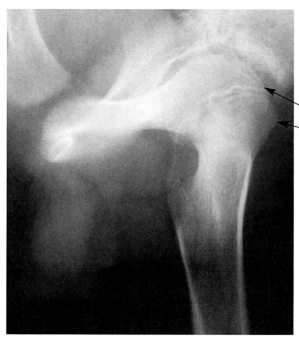

Loss of alignment of epiphysis and metaphysis; epiphysis has slipped posteriorly and inferiorly = slipped capital femoral epiphysis

Lateral view

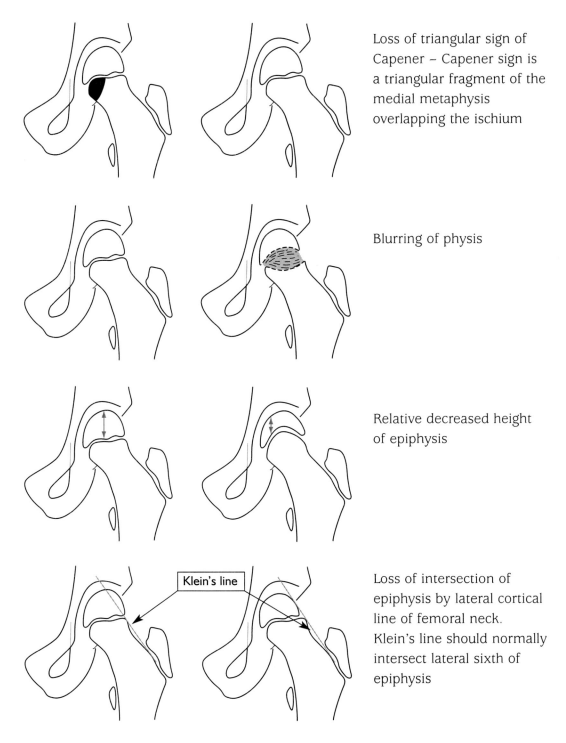

Loss of triangular sign of Capener – Capener sign is a triangular fragment of the medial metaphysis overlapping the ischium

Blurring of physis

Relative decreased height of epiphysis

Klein's line

Loss of intersection of epiphysis by lateral cortical line of femoral neck. Klein's line should normally intersect lateral sixth of epiphysis

Figure 9.1
Radiographic findings in slipped capital femoral epiphysis (normal on the left)

Case 77

Patient was knocked off bicycle, now has pain in hip.

Describe the radiograph.

What are some of the complications of this injury?

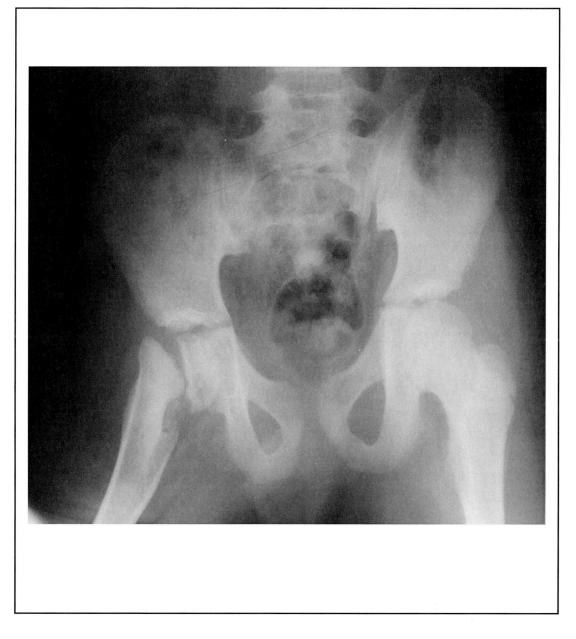

Answer to Case 77

There is a slipped femoral epiphysis of the right hip. If the patient is not treated then exuberant callus will form on the superolateral aspect of the slip forming what is called 'Herndon's hump'. Due to the precarious blood supply to the hip, slipped epiphysis may lead to avascular necrosis (in 25 per cent of patients). Other complications are chondrolysis (in about 30 to 35 per cent of patients), which occurs within one year of slippage and may be evident by gradual narrowing of the joint space. Early arthritic changes are also a complication. Pins are normally inserted following such a slip under image intensifier control.

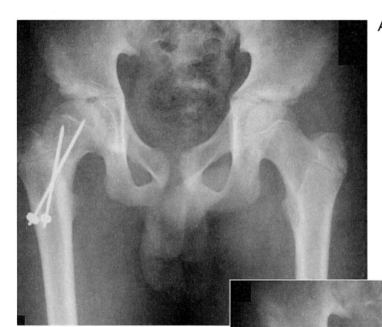

Anterior posterior view

Frog lateral view

Case 78

Adolescent fell during school sports day. Now has a painful right hip.

Can you see an injury, before viewing the lateral radiograph overpage?

What is the name of the accessory ossicle sometimes found here?

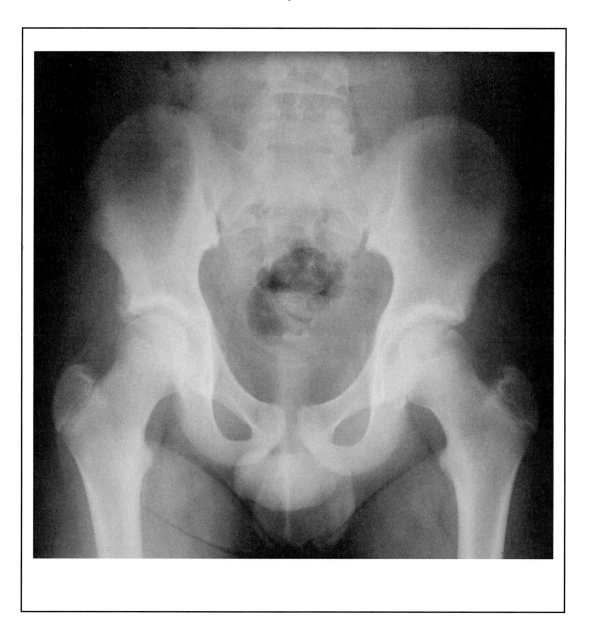

Answer to Case 78

There is an avulsion from the anterior iliac spine. If both hips are compared it will be seen that there is no such area on the left hip. However there is a normal accessory ossicle sometimes found here called the os acetabulum. Accessory ossicles are normally well corticated and rounded (difficult to assess this on the pelvis radiograph). The lateral radiograph demonstrates the bony fragment anterior to the acetabulum, confirming it is an avulsion not an accessory ossicle. Notice the normal triradiate cartilage of the acetabulum on these radiographs.

Lateral view of right hip

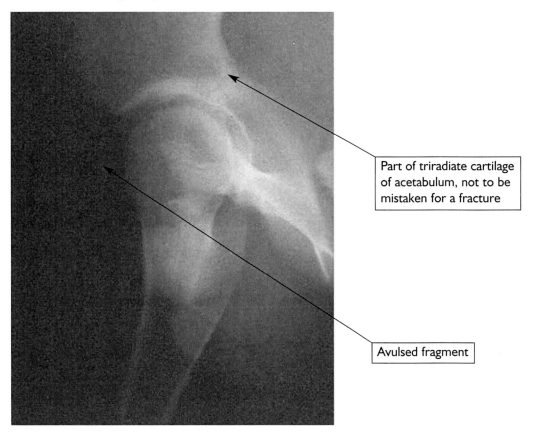

Part of triradiate cartilage of acetabulum, not to be mistaken for a fracture

Avulsed fragment

Case 79

Cheerleader fell awkwardly, now painful left hip.

Describe the radiographs.

Is there an injury? If so, what ligament is involved?

In what age group do these injuries of the pelvis commonly occur?

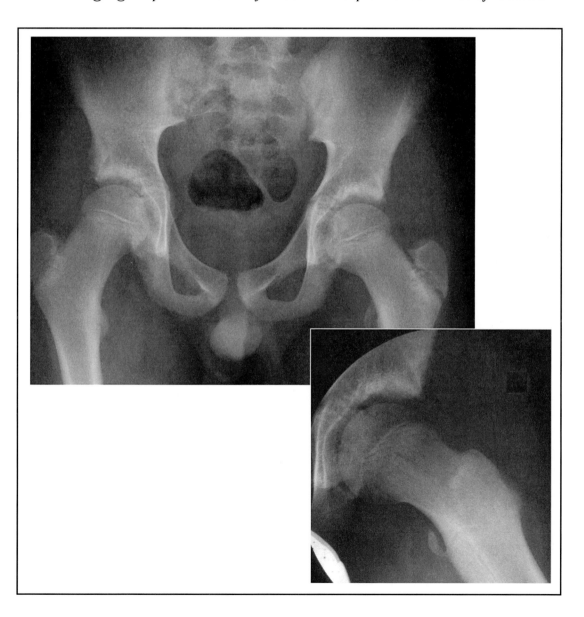

Answer to Case 79

There is an avulsion of the left lesser trochanter of the left hip (compare one side to the other). Avulsions of the apophyses of the pelvis are common between 12 to 16 years of age. They commonly occur in long-jumpers, sprinters, gymnasts and cheerleaders. The ligament involved in this case is the iliopsoas. Figure 9.2 shows the avulsions of the apophyses that may occur in the pelvis and their attached ligaments. The apophyses are weaker than the ligaments, hence are avulsed during trauma; the same injury occurring in an adult would probably result in tearing of the ligament. Remember the apophyses of the pelvis are the last to fuse at 25 years of age, so potentially avulsions may occur until this age.

One of the most commonly avulsed apophyses is at the ischial tuberosity where the hamstrings attach. When an avulsion occurs here it often lays down lots of bone, which if sufficient can trap the sciatic nerve in later life causing problems sitting down. The gross amount of bone laid down may be mistaken as osteomyelitis or Ewing sarcoma, so care is required – there may not be a history of trauma.

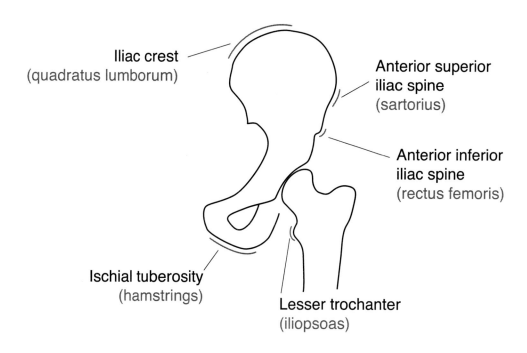

Figure 9.2
Common sites of apophyseal avulsion and muscle attachment

Case 80

Is any injury demonstrated on this radiograph?

Describe Hilgenreiner's line and Perkins' line and their use.

What is the probable cause of the artefacts inferior to the symphysis pubis?

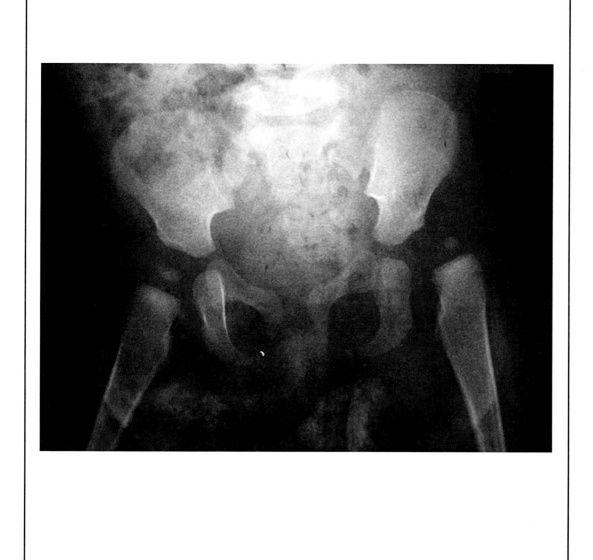

Answer to Case 80

This is an example of developmental dysplasia of the left hip (DDH), previously known as congenital dislocation of the hip.

It is not related to trauma, but very rarely, as in this case, may be found when presenting to the emergency department regarding some other hip problem. It is painless and may be detected at birth when a baby is checked prior to discharge, or later because of asymmetrical skin creases or leg-length discrepancy or waddling gait (if bilateral).

Hilgenreiner's line is a line drawn from one triradiate cartilage to the other triradiate cartilage; Perkins' line is a line drawn inferior from the anterior inferior iliac spine. The femoral epiphysis should lie in the inner lower quadrant formed by these lines. If the femoral epiphysis is superior to Hilgenreiner's line, it is superior subluxed; if it is lateral to Perkins' line, it is laterally subluxed; if both, it is dislocated. Hence in Figure 9.3 the right hip is laterally subluxed, the left hip is dislocated.

The artefact seen on the pelvis is the baby's nappy. This is very distracting and can hide abnormalities so patients should not have pelvic x-rays with a nappy on.

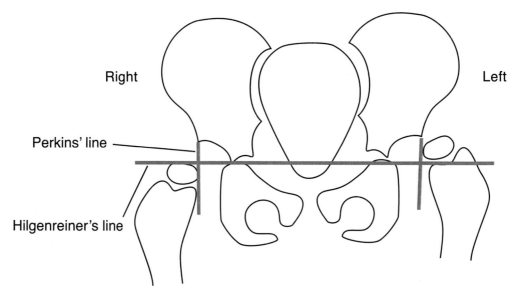

Figure 9.3
Developmental dysplasia of the hip

Another case of developmental dysplasia of the hip is shown below.

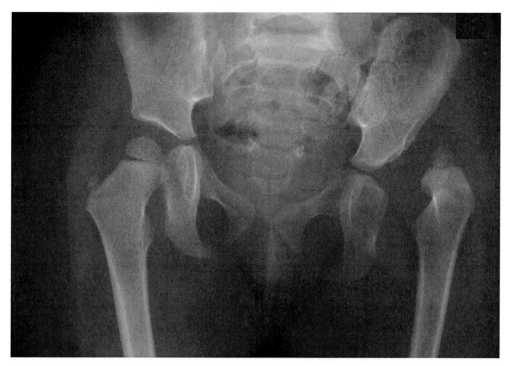

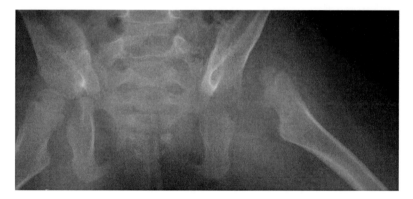

If you draw Hilgenreiner's and Perkins' line the left hip is dislocated (see anterior posterior image, top). The frog lateral hip (shown above) confirms this, but perhaps was unnecessary as the injury is demonstrated adequately on the pelvis radiograph. The left femoral epiphysis is smaller than the right; this often occurs in developmental dysplasia of the hip and is a secondary phenomenon along with a shallow acetabulum fossa.

Case 81

Patient with cerebral palsy has less movement than normal in right hip.

Describe the radiograph.

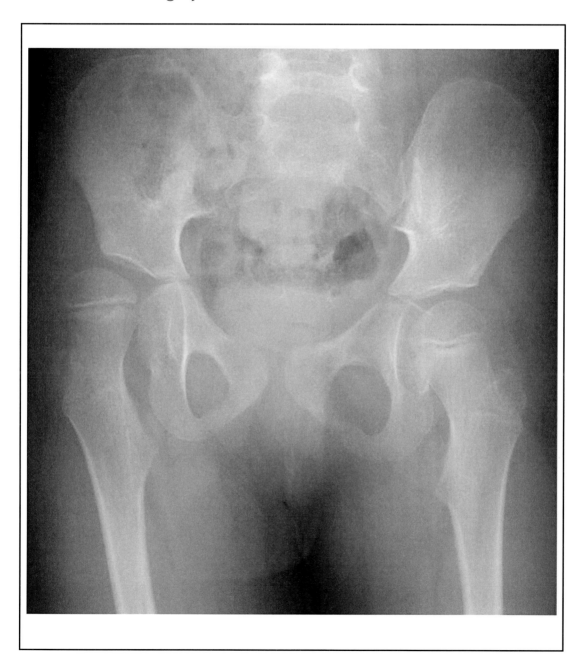

Answer to Case 81

Patients with cerebral palsy are prone to fractures (whilst being moved by carers, due to disuse osteoporosis); however in this case no fracture can be detected. The right hip has moved laterally and superiorly (remember Hilgenreiner's line and Perkins' line). The right hip has a migration index of 50 per cent; this is likely to be chronic and likely to be painless.

Case 82

Patient was involved in a road traffic incident.

Describe the radiograph.

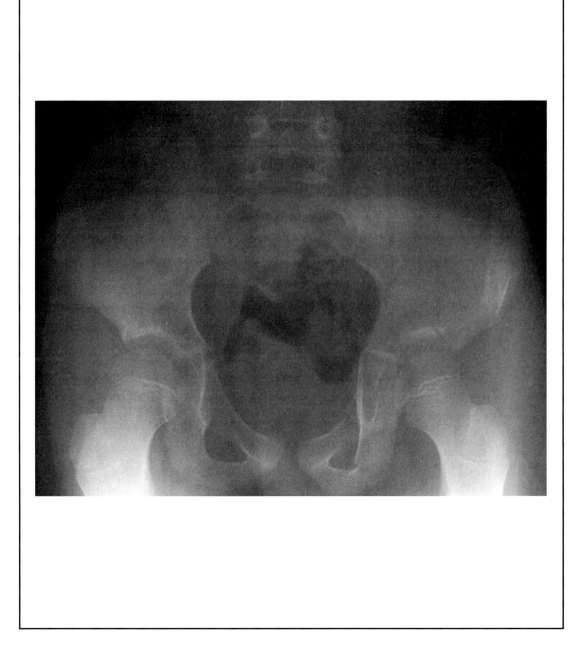

Answer to Case 82

There is a fracture of the left superior pubic ramus and ischial tuberosity. As with adults you should treat the pelvis as a bony ring. If a fracture of the bony ring is identified in one place, look carefully for another. Especially if you see a fracture anteriorly, look at the posterior pelvis and acetabulum area. Remember that Tile and Pennal (1980) divide pelvic fractures into three main mechanisms of injury; lateral compression, anterior compression and vertical shear. The most common mechanism of injury is lateral compression (see p. 202 for a summary of each mechanism of injury). On the left side there is a lucent line in the acetabular roof, and compared to the right hemipelvis the medial acetabulum appears to bulge into the pelvic inlet (there is disruption of the left iliopubic line), indicative of an acetabulum fracture; computerised axial tomography confirmed this. A Judet view was performed, as shown on p. 252, but this is not conclusive concerning the acetabular fracture. Judet views are used to demonstrate acetabular fractures; two oblique views centred on the symptomatic hip, one with 45 degrees medial tilt, one with 45 degrees lateral tilt, are performed.

Remember when assessing children's pelvic radiographs that the sacroiliac joints (S.I. joints) are wider than in an adult, as is the width of the symphysis pubis (2.5 cm in an adult). This is due to the cartilage at these sites, which is not radiographically demonstrated. Also remember not to mistake the triradiate cartilage of the acetabulum for a fracture.

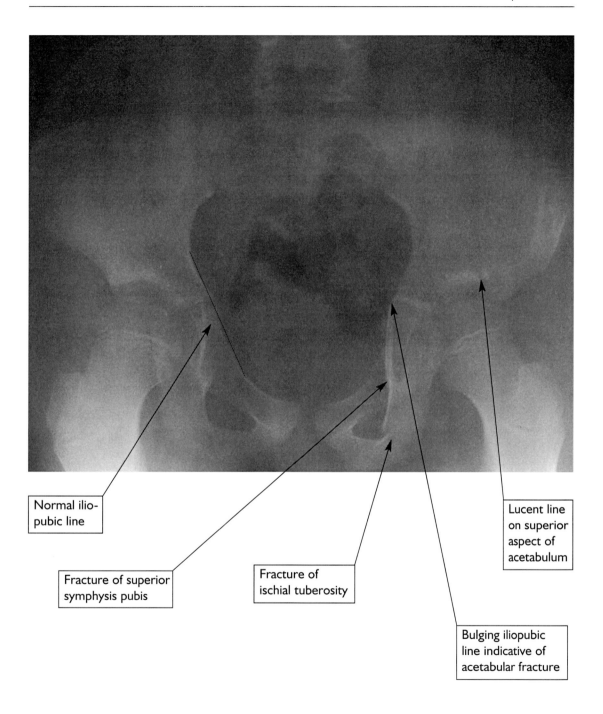

Normal ilio-pubic line

Fracture of superior symphysis pubis

Fracture of ischial tuberosity

Bulging iliopubic line indicative of acetabular fracture

Lucent line on superior aspect of acetabulum

Judet's view

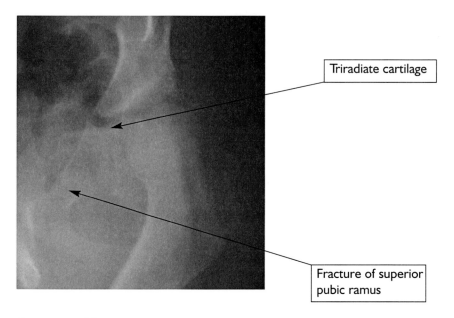

Triradiate cartilage

Fracture of superior pubic ramus

Features of *lateral* compression injuries
- Most common bilateral fractures of the superior and inferior pubic rami in the coronal plane.
- Sacral alar fracture impacted.
- Sacroiliac ligaments (both anterior and posterior) remain intact.
- Severe compression may disrupt the posterior ligament complex.

Features of *anterior* compression injuries
- Results in diastasis of the pubis and sacro-iliac joints.
- Less than 2.5 cm (adults) widening of the symphysis pubis leaves the sacroiliac joints intact.
- More than 2.5 cm (adults) widening of the symphysis pubis is accompanied by disruption of the anterior ligaments of the sacroiliac joints.

Features of *vertical shear* injuries
- Forces transmitted by the femur to the acetabulum result in vertical displacement of the ipsilateral pelvis.
- Results in fracture of the ipsilateral sacral alar and pubic ramus.
- The posterior sacroiliac ligament complex is disrupted, making the injury unstable.

Case 83

Patient was involved in a road traffic incident.

Describe the injury.

When reviewing a fracture of the mid shaft of the femur, is there any area you should be concerned about?

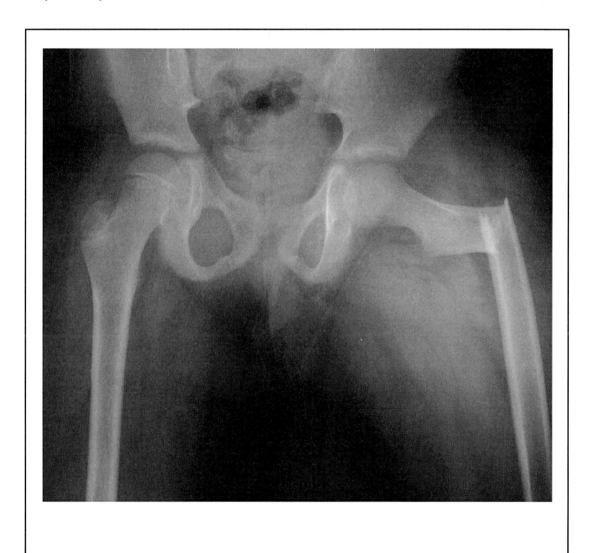

Answer to Case 83

There is a fracture of the left femur proximal third, with foreshortening and lateral angulation of the proximal femur, by about 90 degrees. When there is severe angulation of a fracture of the shaft of the femur concerns should be raised as to whether the hip has dislocated (see Figure 9.4). In this case the epiphysis of the femur does not appear to be in normal alignment with the acetabulum, although the width of the joint space appears normal, hence it is probably not dislocated but requires another view to confirm.

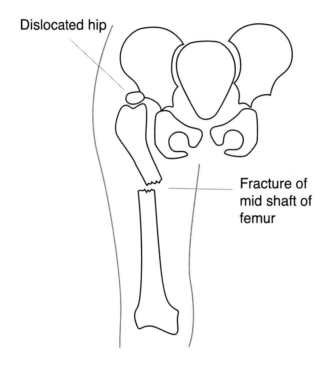

Figure 9.4
Fracture of mid shaft of femur, with associated dislocated hip

Case 84

Patient has pain in hip.

Describe the radiograph.

Describe how you evaluate for a joint effusion of a hip on a pelvic radiograph.

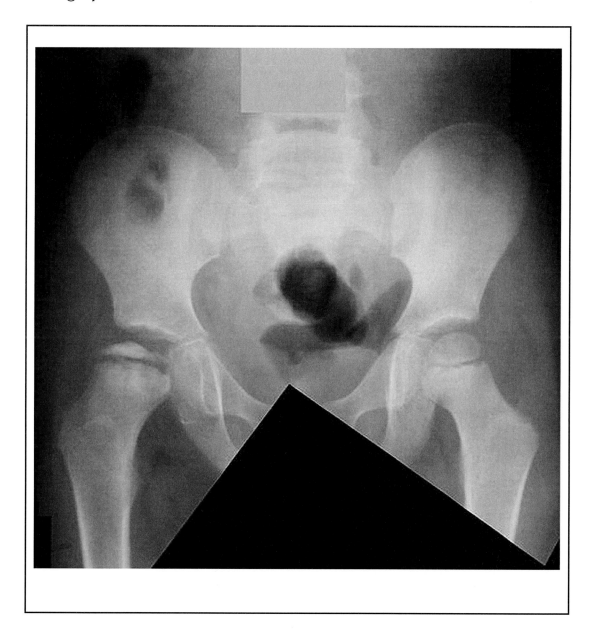

Answer to Case 84

There is a right hip joint effusion demonstrated by the increased distance between the radiographic teardrop and the metaphysis of the femur compared to the left (see below). Ultrasound is more sensitive for detecting hip effusions.

The right epiphysis is smaller and denser than the left. The right physeal plate is irregular with lucent areas in the metaphysis. The right hip is slightly laterally subluxed (remember to use Perkins' line; see case 80) – this is called Waldenström's sign. This has the radiographic appearance of Legg–Calvé–Perthes disease (often referred to as Perthes disease). It commonly occurs in males between the ages of 3 and twelve years of age, and is bilateral in 10 per cent of cases. The onset may be insidious or sudden. The symptoms are worsened by activity and relieved by rest. It is a self-limiting disease of 2 to 6 years' duration.

The appearances of the right femur are not acute (stage two of Perthes disease); why the patient has exacerbated pain and effusion needs further investigation.

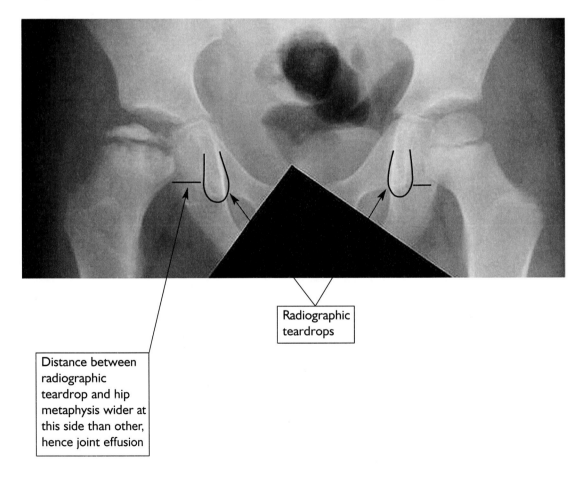

Radiographic teardrops

Distance between radiographic teardrop and hip metaphysis wider at this side than other, hence joint effusion

Case 85

This young adult has longstanding hip problems.

Describe the radiograph.

What disease process is the most likely cause of this appearance?

Comment on the different stages of this disease and their radiographic appearance.

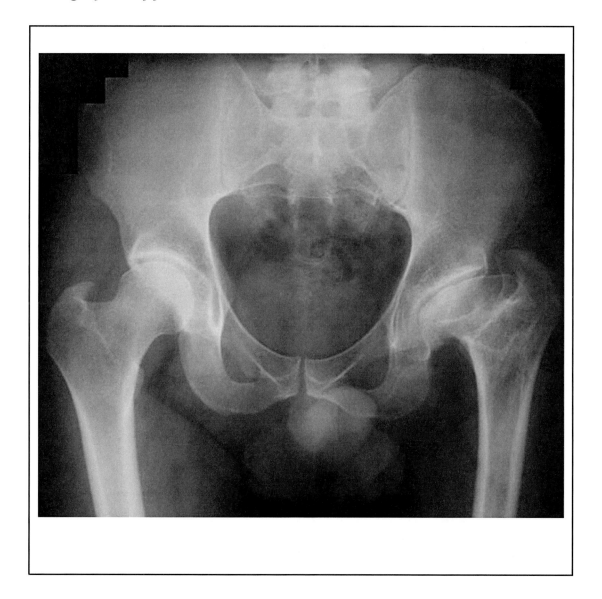

Answer to Case 85

There is a flattened left femoral head (mushroom deformity) with a short broad femoral neck (coxa magna). This is the typical appearance of the fourth and end stage of Legg–Calvé–Perthes disease. Below are described the four stages of the disease and their radiographic appearance.

Stage one is the avascular stage. The radiographic appearance is joint effusion (widening of teardrop distance) and lateral displacement of the head of femur (Waldenström's sign).

Stage two is the necrotic stage. Radiographically the earliest bony appearance is a radiolucent line (crescent sign) in the subchondral bone closest to the articular surface; frog lateral radiographs of the hips are helpful in visualising this. There is increased density of the epiphysis, sometimes referred to as 'snowy cap'; radiolucent areas will develop within the femoral epiphysis (which represent areas of necrotic bone that are undergoing demineralisation). As the disease progresses the epiphysis becomes irregular, fragmented and flattened (collapsed). See Case 84 which is in this phase.

Stage three is the healing stage. Dead tissue is replaced by new bone.

Stage four is the end stage. Radiographically there is usually a flattened femoral epiphysis (mushroom deformity) and a short broad femoral neck (coxa magna). There may be enlargement of the acetabulum to accommodate the abnormal femoral head – coxa plana – (flattened femoral head), coxa magna (broad femoral head and neck) and coxa valga or vara. Early degenerative changes of the affected hip are common. Coxa valga is an increased neck shaft angle of more than 135 degrees; coxa vara is a reduced neck shaft angle of less than 120 degrees.

10.

Spine, skull and facial trauma

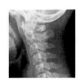

Case 86

Patient in car seat in a car involved in a collision.

Describe the radiographs.

Comment on the differing radiographic appearances of vascular markings and skull fractures.

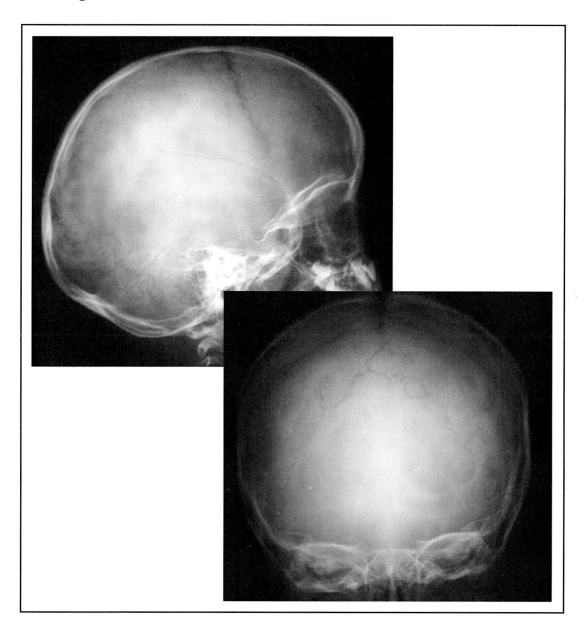

Answer to Case 86

There is a simple linear fracture of the parietal bone, demonstrated only on the lateral radiograph. The additional importance of identifying this fracture is that the middle meningeal artery lies in this region and may be injured, leading to intracranial bleeding.

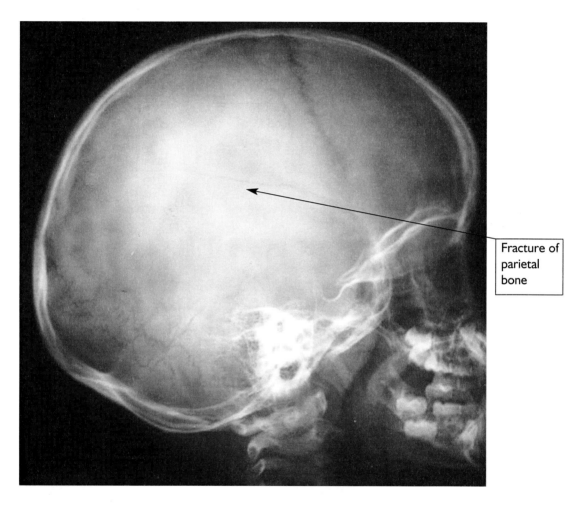

Fracture of parietal bone

Vascular markings on skull radiographs may be mistaken for fractures. In general fractures of the skull appear densely black (this is due to both the inner and outer tables being involved), do not taper or have branches that taper, and do not have sclerotic margins. Vascular markings, however, appear grey on radiographs (as vessels lie in grooves and in the inner table of the skull), have branches that decrease in size, and have sclerotic margins.

Sutures and accessory sutures may be mistaken for fractures. Hence it is imperative to know the position of the normal sutures and the likely position of the accessory sutures, to prevent misdiagnosis (see Case 87 for more on the position of sutures). The concern is not to overlook or incorrectly diagnose a non-accidental injury (see Chapter 1). It is also common to see one or several wormian bones on paediatric skull radiographs. Intra-sutural bone (a wormian bone) is a small area of the skull, normally 1–2 cm in diameter, completely surrounded by a suture.

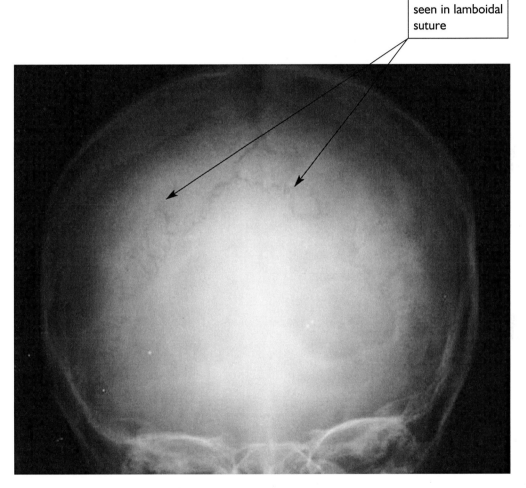

Wormian bones seen in lamboidal suture

These days it is rare to perform an x-ray of the skull apart from as part of a skeletal survey, or if there is a suspected foreign body (FB). However, we still should know the anatomy of the skull and be able to identify a fracture, as I have x-rayed an adult patient for suspected FB and found an underlying depressed skull fracture.

CT is now normally carried out in preference to x-rays (see the NICE Clinical Guidelines 176, issued in January 2014, Head injury: Triage, assessment, investigation and early management of head injury in children, young people and adults). The guidelines comment that 'head injury is the commonest cause of death and disability in people aged 1–40 years in the UK. Each year 1.4 million people attend A&E in England and Wales with a head injury; between 33% and 50% are children under 16 years of age'. X-rays of the skull may or may not demonstrate a fracture. However, regardless of whether or not there is a fracture, there may be an intercranial bleed, and it is this that leads to mortality and requires a CT scan to visualise – hence the recommendation for CT rather than skull x-ray. The NICE guidelines give clear advice on when a CT should be performed.

For children who have sustained a head injury and have any of the following risk factors, a CT should be performed within 1 hour:

- Suspicion of NAI
- Post-traumatic seizure, but no history of epilepsy
- On initial examination, Glasgow coma scale (GCS) less than 14; in children under one year, less than 15
- At 2 hours after injury, GCS less than 15
- Suspected open or depressed fracture
- Any sign of basal skull fracture
- Focal neurological deficit
- For children under one year, presence of bruise, swelling or laceration of more than 5cm on the head.

For children who have sustained a head injury and have more than one of the following risk factors, a CT should be performed within 1 hour:

- Loss of consciousness for more than 5 minutes
- Abnormal drowsiness
- Three or more discrete episodes of vomiting
- Dangerous mechanism of injury
- Amnesia.

The NICE guidelines comment that 25–30 per cent of children under 2 years of age who are hospitalised with head injury have an abusive head injury and will therefore go on to have a skeletal survey (see Chapter 1). The guidelines hence suggest that a clinician with training in safeguarding should be involved in the initial assessment of any paediatric patient in A&E (although everyone who works in the NHS has mandatory safeguarding training to different levels, depending on their role).

Today the patient in this case would have had a CT scan for such a significant injury, not an x-ray. This is why most of the skull x-ray cases have been replaced in this second edition.

Case 87

Describe the radiographs.

Comment on the position of the normal sutures. Name the additional sutures that may be found in a paediatric skull.

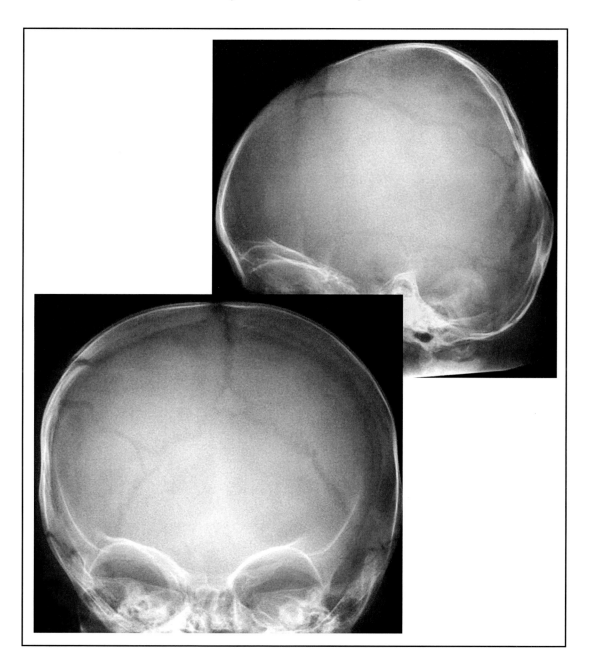

Answer to Case 87

The initial report read: 'there is a lucent line across the right parietal bone from the coronal suture to the lamboid suture. It takes a wavy course and appears to bifurcate posteriorly. The overall appearances are possibly more in keeping with a unilateral intraparietal suture than a fracture.) A similar appearance is seen in Keats' book – see reading list – normal variants that may simulate disease. However, another more senior radiologist's final report read: 'there is a step in the outline of the skull vault on the anterior posterior view and I think this appearance is due to a fracture of the parietal bone rather than a subparietal suture'. This demonstrates what a difficult diagnosis a skull fracture is in a child.

In paediatrics, differentiating a skull fracture from a normal accessory suture can sometimes be very difficult; a sound knowledge of sites of the normal sutures and most common accessory sutures is helpful.

The normal sutures found on skull radiographs are the sagittal, coronal, lamboidal, squamosal, occipitomastoid (Figures 10.1–10.2). Common accessory sutures are the metopic suture (the commonest, which may persist into adulthood, divides frontal bone into two halves), the accessory parietal suture (may be incomplete, vertical, horizontal or oblique), the mendosal suture (extends posteriorly from the lamboidal suture on lateral view, and passes medially on Towne's view) and the innominate suture (always present in infants but disappears as the child matures). See Figures 10.3–10.5.

The NICE guidelines (2003) for assessment and management of head injury advocate that skull films are only needed where there is suspicion of non-accidental injury or where CT is not available, and children need a period of observation. Hence we are seeing fewer skull x-rays and some of the cases in this chapter are old and would today have CT instead.

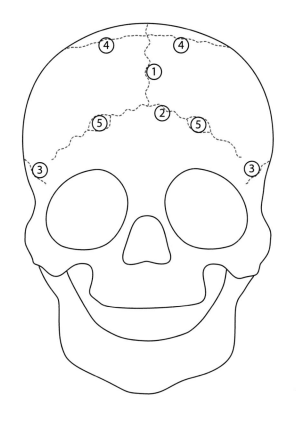

Figure 10.1
Normal sutures on anterior posterior radiograph

1 Sagittal suture

2 Lamboidal suture

3 Squamosal suture

4 Coronal suture

5 Wormian bone

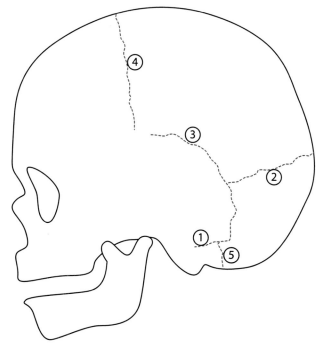

Figure 10.2
Normal sutures on lateral radiograph

1 Occipitomastoid suture

2 Lamboidal suture

3 Squamousal suture

4 Coronal suture

5 Innominate suture

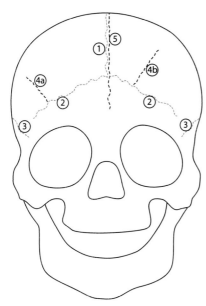

Figure 10.3

Possible positions of accessory sutures on anterior posterior radiograph

1 Sagittal suture

2 Lamboidal suture

3 Squamosal suture

4a Accessory parietal suture

4b Accessory parietal suture

5 Metopic suture

Figure 10.4

Possible positions of parietal accessory sutures on lateral radiograph

1 Occipitomastoid suture

2 Lamboidal suture

3 Squamosal suture

4 Coronal suture

5 Innominate suture

A A complete horizontal accessory parietal suture

B, C Incomplete accessory parietal sutures

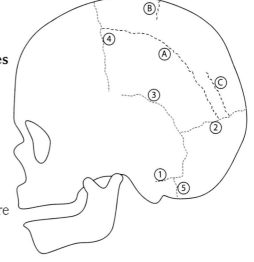

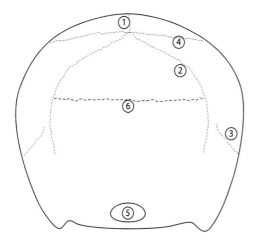

Figure 10.5 **Accessory sutures on a Towne's radiograph**

1 Sagittal suture

2 Lamboidal suture

3 Squamosal suture

4 Coronal suture

5 Foramen magnum

6 Mendosal suture (occasionally it is complete as demonstrated here, but more often it is incomplete)

Case 88

Patient fell from climbing frame onto chin. Query fracture of mandible?

Write a provisional image evaluation.

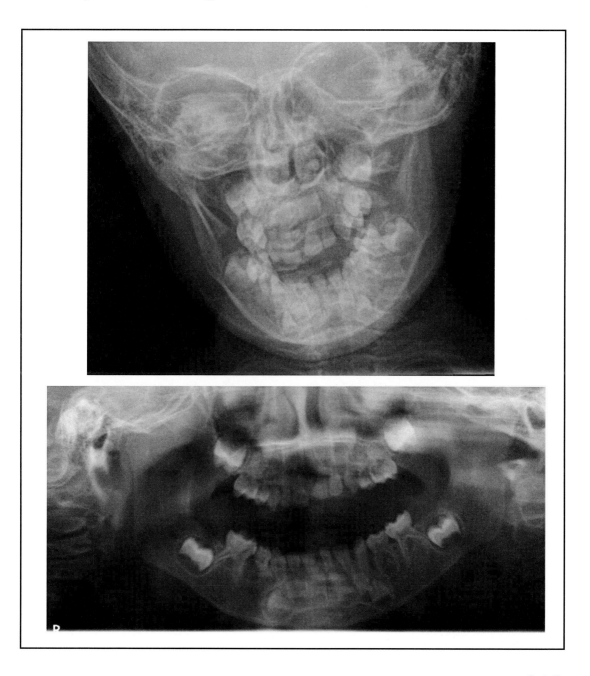

Answer to Case 88

There is no bony injury. In this age group, it is sometimes difficult to obtain good-quality images so extra care is required when reviewing the images. Look especially for condylar fractures and parasymphysis fractures (the latter being difficult to detect), although fractures of the mandible are rare in this age group.

Case 89

Patient was involved in a road traffic collision.

Write a provisional image evaluation.

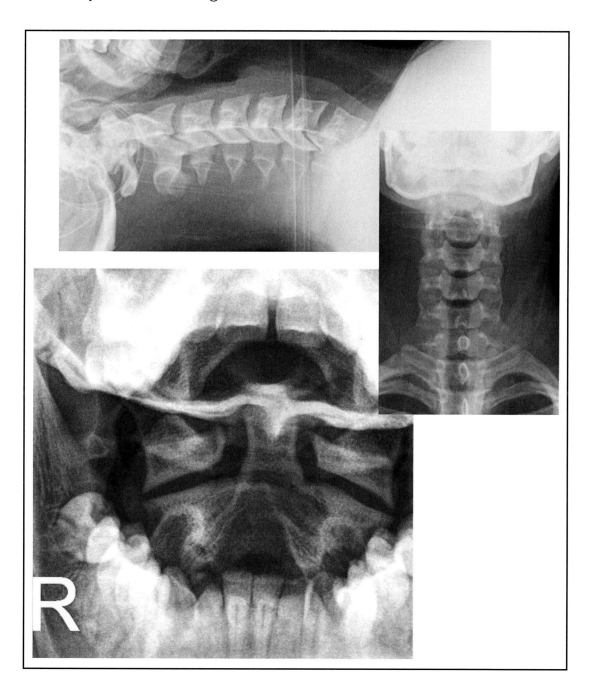

Answer to Case 89

Cervical vertebra 7 and thoracic vertebra 1 are not clearly demonstrated. However, there is no acute bony injury demonstrated. Normal vertebral height and alignment are maintained, and there are normal prevertebral soft tissues. Be careful not to mistake the normal ring apophysis of the vertebra as fractures. Also be aware of normal variants of the odontoid peg, such as os terminale and os odontoideum (see diagram below and see Cases 91 and 92 for further information).

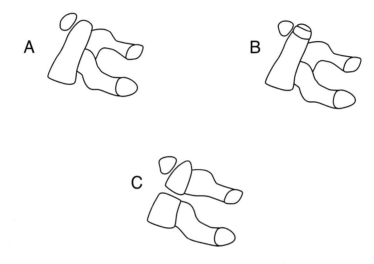

Figure 10.6 **Spectrum of os terminale variants**
A – normal fusion
B – a simple unfused os terminale
C – os odontoideum (a result of overgrown os terminale)

Case 90

Patient was involved in a road traffic collision.

Write a provisional image evaluation.

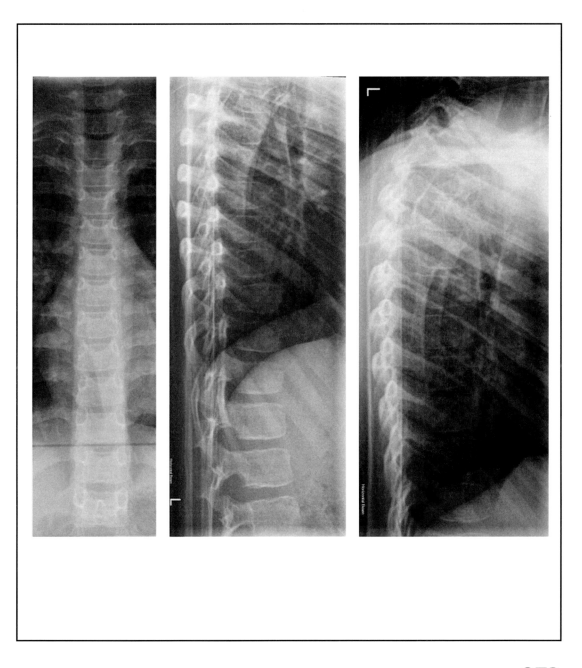

Answer to Case 90

There is no acute bony injury; normal vertebral alignment and height is maintained. Again, be aware of ring apophysis of the vertebra. As with adults, look very carefully at thoracic vertebra 12 and lumbar vertebra 1, as this is where most of the injuries occur.

Case 91

Patient was in a road traffic incident, now pain in neck. Lateral cervical spine x-ray was performed in the resuscitation room.

Discuss the radiograph and findings (if any).

Discuss the pre-vertebral soft tissues in children compared to adults.

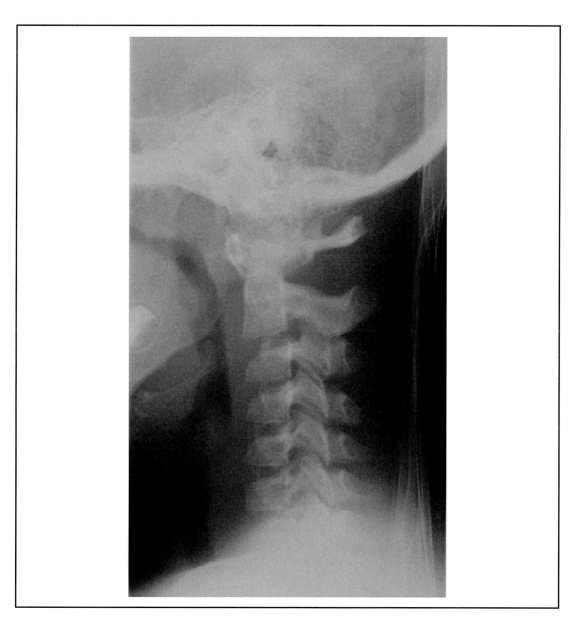

Answer to Case 91

The intervertebral disc space between cervical C7 and dorsal D1 is not adequately demonstrated on this radiograph. This area always needs to be included on a trauma cervical spine whether it be adult or child as this is a common area of injury. There is loss of lordosis which may be due to muscle spasm. There is a slight offset anteriorly at cervical vertebrae C2 and C3. The fulcrum of flexion in adults is cervical vertebrae C5 and C6, whereas in a child it is cervical vertebrae C2/C3. In a young child this may result in a physiological anterior offset of cervical vertebra two on three being visualised on the radiograph; occasionally a similar offset may occur at cervical vertebrae C3/C4. This offset can sometimes be seen up to the age of 30 and should not be mistaken for a fracture. Flexion and extension radiographs were undertaken, which demonstrate the anterior offset even more on the flexion radiograph, but normal alignment is demonstrated on the extension radiograph.

It is debatable whether these flexion and extension radiographs should have been taken, considering the young age of the patient, and that the original radiograph is normal, i.e. no evidence of trauma. We must often balance the risk of missing a spinal injury against exposure to extra radiation. Perhaps in this case there were neurological signs that warranted extra views.

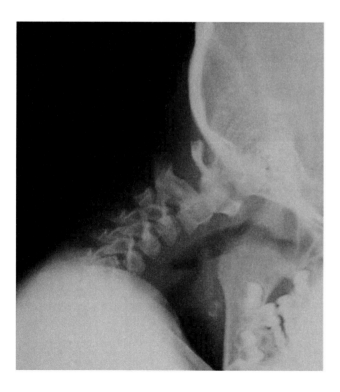

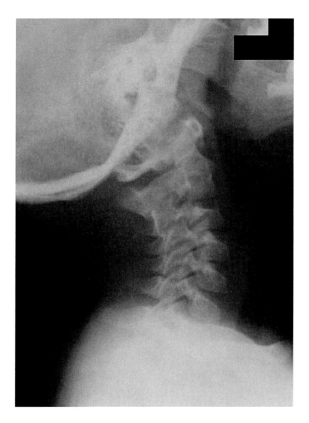

The pre-vertebral soft tissues in adults should not be greater than 5 mm at cervical level C3 and C4, and less than 22 mm at cervical vertebra C6; greater distances than this are indicative of effusion and cervical injury. In children the distances are different; the pre-vertebral soft tissue should be two-thirds the width of the body of C2 at the C3/4 level and not more than 14 mm at C6.

Inherent elasticity in the paediatric cervical spine can allow severe spinal cord injury to occur in the absence of x-ray findings. This is called SCIWORA syndrome – Spinal Cord Syndrome WithOut Radiological Abnormality. In this case magnetic resonance imaging (MRI) is helpful.

The features of SCIWORA were first defined in 1982 by Pang and Wilerger as 'objective signs of myelopathy as a result of trauma with no evidence of fracture or ligamentous instability on plain spine radiographs'. Delayed onset of SCIWORA in children as late as 4 days post injury has been documented.

Case 92

Patient was involved in a road traffic accident. Radiographs were taken in the resuscitation room.

Is there a fracture present?

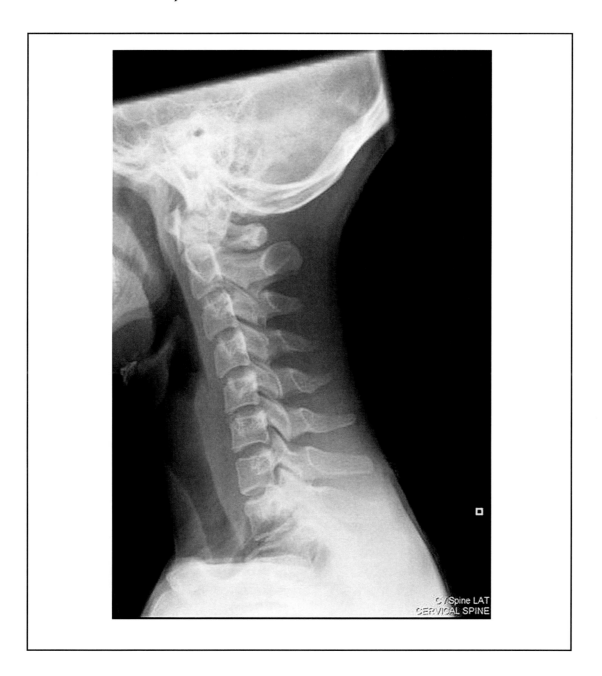

C/Spine LAT
CERVICAL SPINE

Answer to Case 92

There is no fracture present. On the anteroinferior border of cervical vertebra bodies C3 to C6 can be seen the ring apophyses of the vertebral bodies, not to be mistaken for fractures. Again there is slight offset at cervical vertebrae C3/C4 (as discussed in Case 91) and loss of lordosis. The anterior posterior and peg views taken later demonstrated no injury. As the patient later revealed no clinical signs of neck injury, the clinicians concluded there was no cervical spine injury.

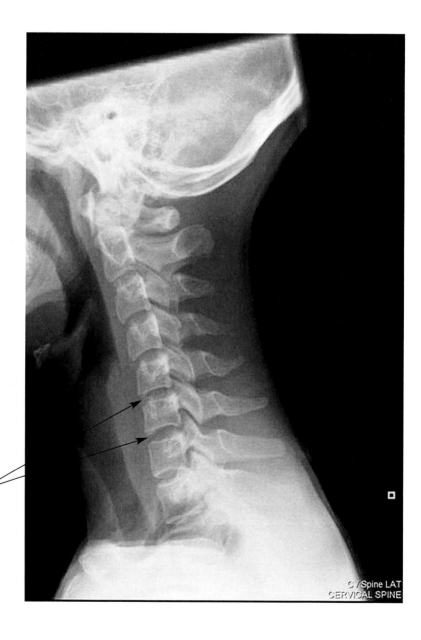

Ring apophysis

C/Spine LAT
CERVICAL SPINE

Case 93

This 15-year-old was involved in a fight, receiving a blow to the left side of the face.

Is there an injury?

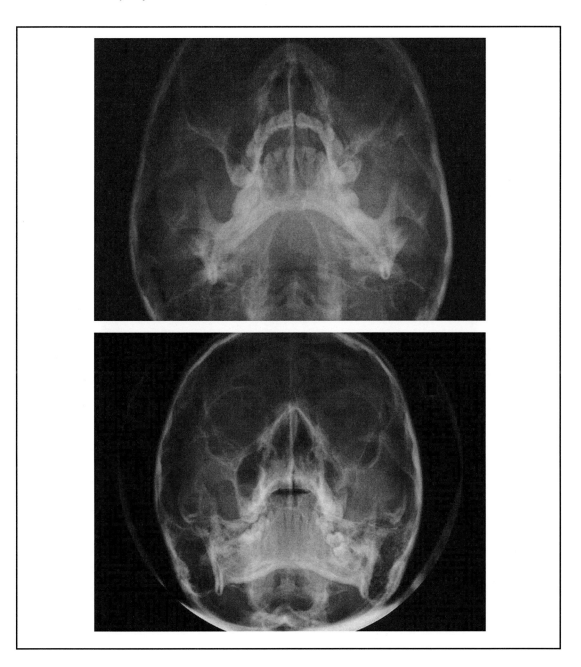

Answer to Case 93

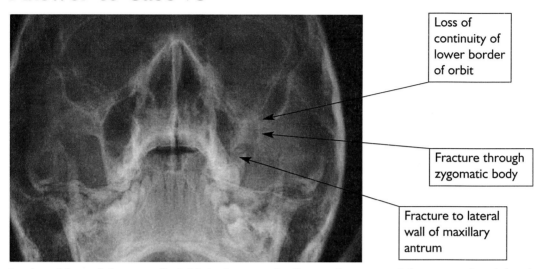

Loss of continuity of lower border of orbit

Fracture through zygomatic body

Fracture to lateral wall of maxillary antrum

In the older adolescent, facial injuries are similar to those in adults. As with adults, look for fluid levels or loss of air in the maxillary antra, as a clue to injury of the facial bones.

A common fracture of the facial bones in an adult is what used to be called a tripod fracture, involving widening of the zygomatico-frontal suture, fracture of the zygomatic arch, and a fracture through the zygomatic body. This is now called the zygomatico maxillary complex fractures (ZMC), as there may be more than the three fractures mentioned. This case has three fractures but only one of the above mentioned in tripod fractures (the fracture of the zygomatic body).

The others are: fracture of the left orbital floor and lateral wall of the left maxillary sinus. This highlights the fact that, when you see one fracture in the face, you should look for others.

Mcgrigor's lines are useful when assessing facial trauma, in order to help avoid missing fractures, and ensure an orderly search for injury (see below for a demonstration of Mcgrigor's lines). For more cases and information on adult facial and spinal injuries, please see another book in this series – *Self Assessment of the Axial Skeleton*.

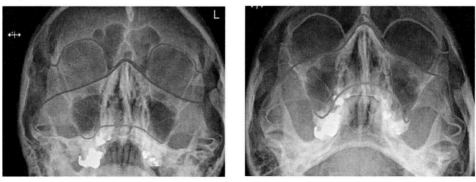

Figure 10.7 **Mcgrigor's lines on OM and OM 30 views**

Case 94

A younger child was hit in the face, resulting in pain and bruising.

Is there an injury?

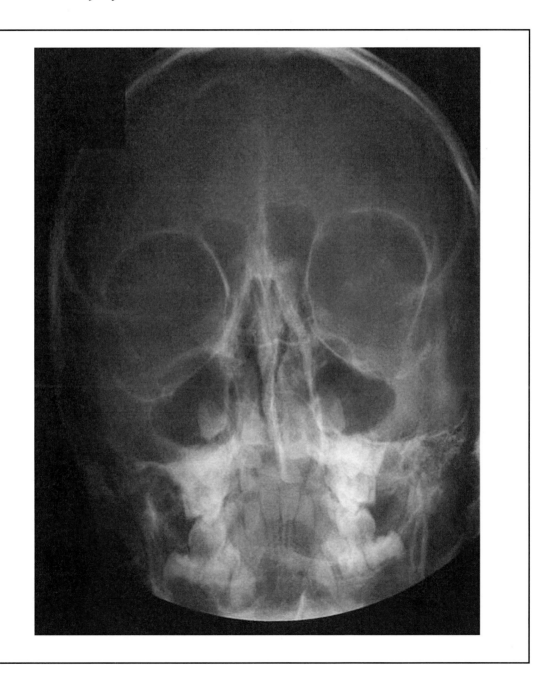

Answer to Case 94

No bony injury was demonstrated. Notice the adult teeth appearing to be in the maxillary antra.

11.

A selection of cases

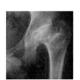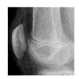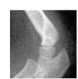

Case 95

Patient thought to have fallen. Is now non-weight bearing with pain on touching leg.

Describe the radiographs.

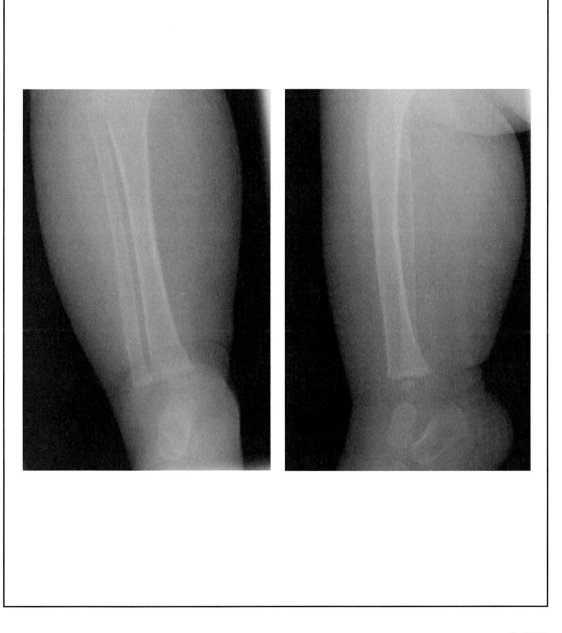

Answer to Case 95

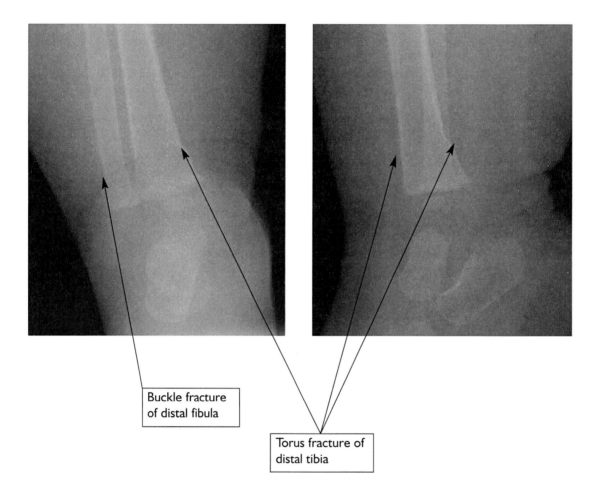

Buckle fracture of distal fibula

Torus fracture of distal tibia

There is a torus fracture of the distal tibia and a buckle fracture of the distal fibula. This highlights the importance of looking carefully at the whole radiograph especially at both bones on tibial and fibular and radial and ulnar radiographs.

Case 96

Patient fell down several steps whilst playing, now unable to weight bear, and pain in ankle.

Describe the radiographs.

Would another view be helpful?

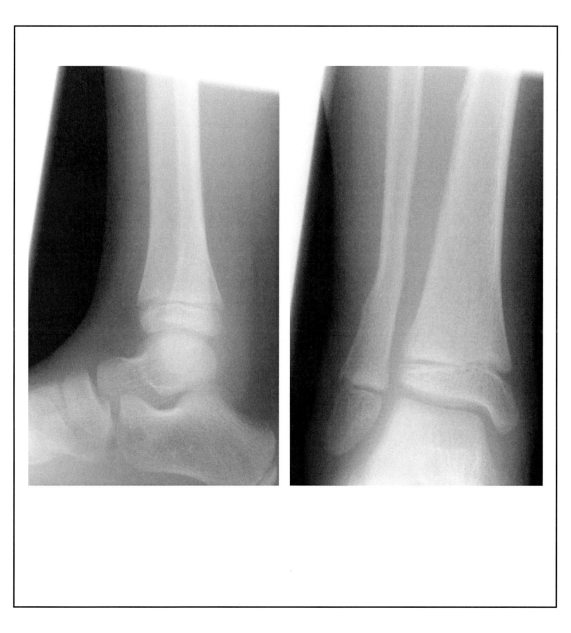

Answer to Case 96

The anterior posterior radiograph demonstrates a sharp lateral angulation of the fibula, typical of a buckle type fracture (see Case 75), but on closer observation a break in the lateral cortex is demonstrated, therefore this is a greenstick fracture. If one fracture is demonstrated check for a second fracture (as mentioned in case 75); there is a break in the cortex of the lateral aspect of the tibia proximal to the fibular fracture – a greenstick fracture. This area is not fully shown on the ankle views and requires full length tibia and fibula radiographs to demonstrate the full extent of the tibial fracture.

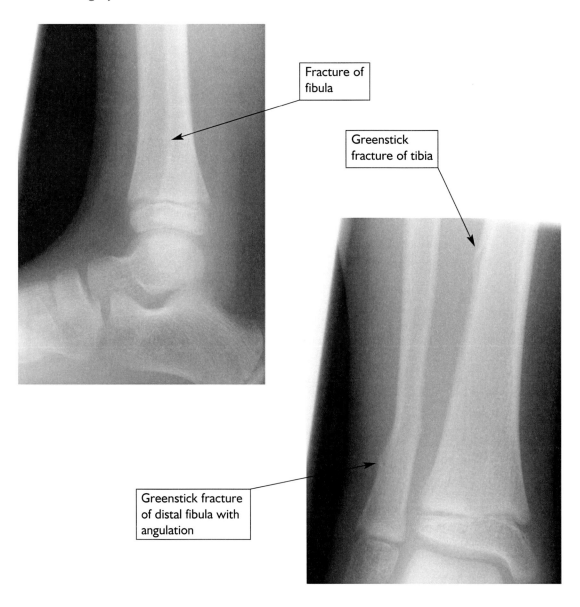

Fracture of fibula

Greenstick fracture of tibia

Greenstick fracture of distal fibula with angulation

Case 97

Patient stubbed toes, now painful toes and metatarsals.

Describe the radiographs.

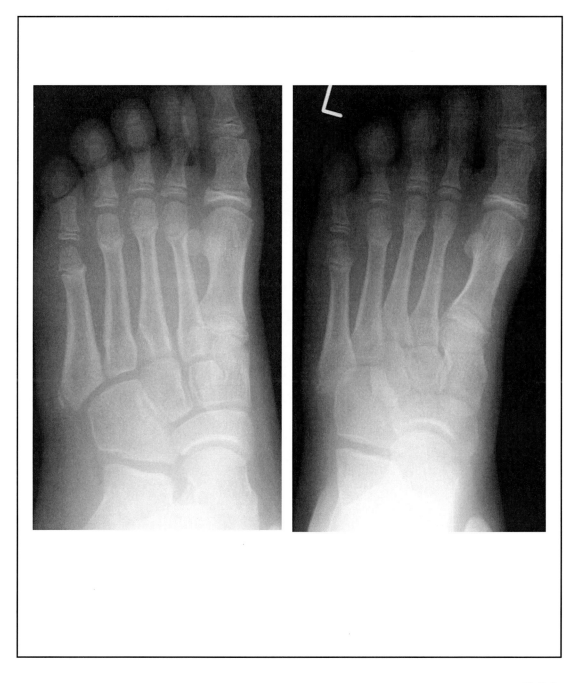

Answer to Case 97

There is a Salter Harris type II fracture of the proximal phalanx of the fourth toe.

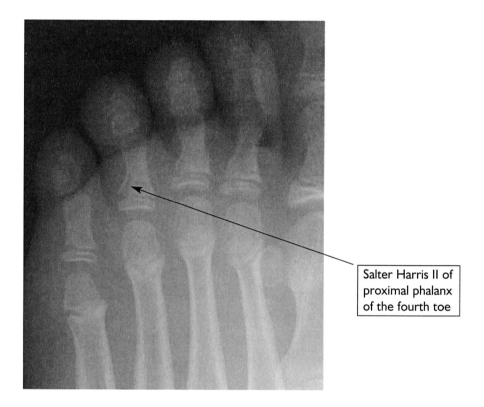

Salter Harris II of proximal phalanx of the fourth toe

Case 98

Patient fell onto outstretched hand, now not using elbow.

Describe the radiographs.

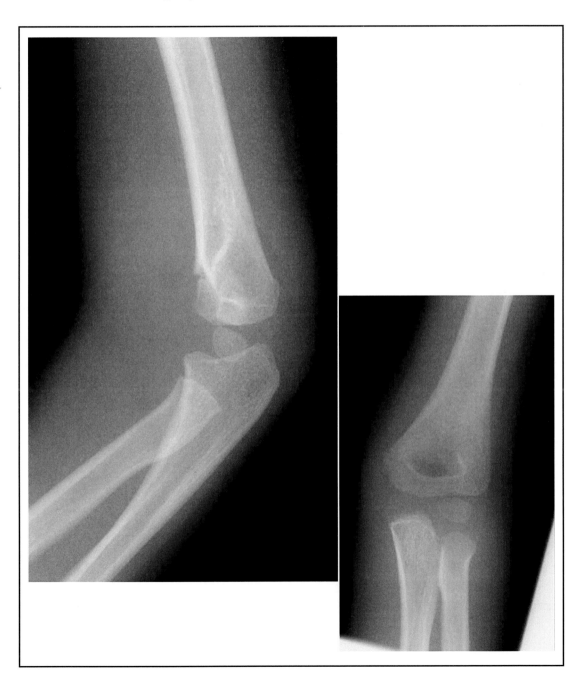

Answer to Case 98

There are raised anterior and posterior fat pads (a joint effusion). The anterior humeral line, instead of passing through the anterior part of the middle third of the capitellum, passes anterior to the capitellum. Both these points are indicative of a supracondylar fracture. There is a fracture demonstrated on the medial and volar aspect of the distal humerus (see Cases 21 and 22).

Case 99

Patient fell, now with pain in clavicle.

Is there an injury?

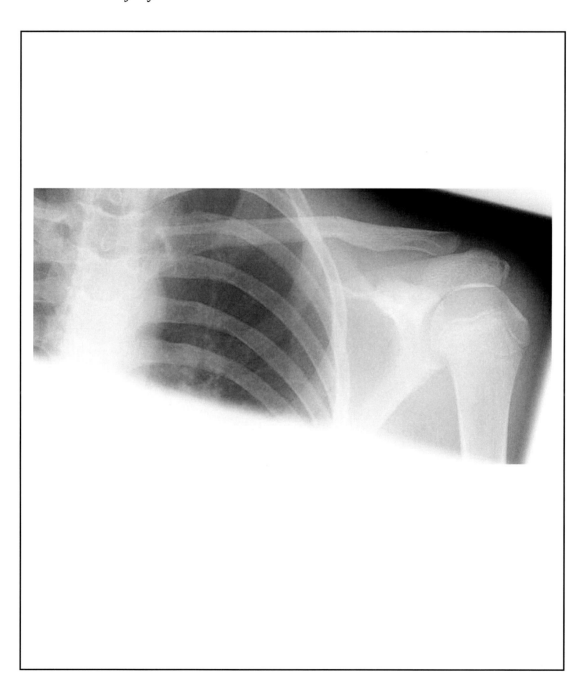

Answer to Case 99

There is a fracture mid shaft of the clavicle. Sometimes this can be a difficult area to visualise radiographically, requiring a cranially angulated radiograph. (See Cases 36 and 38.)

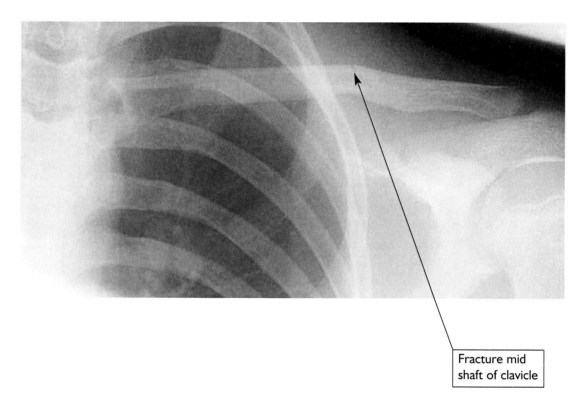

Fracture mid shaft of clavicle

Case 100

Patient fell, inverting ankle, now painful weight-bearing.

Describe the radiographs.

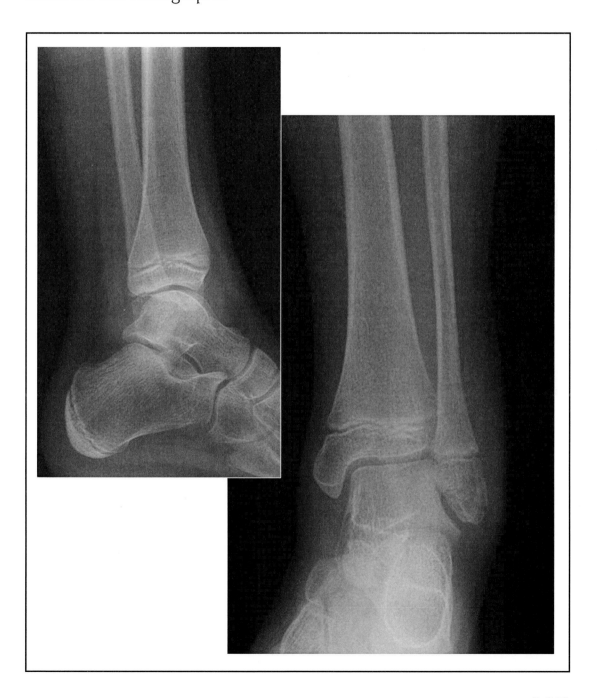

Answer to Case 100

There is a transverse type fracture of the distal fibula (Weber A), with soft tissue swelling. Danis and Weber classified ankle injuries according to the level of the fracture of the fibula. Weber A is a fracture below the ankle joint, Weber B at the joint level (with 50 per cent chance of instability due to involvement of the tibiofibular syndesmosis), and Weber C is a high fibular fracture with instability.

Case 101

Patient fell onto shoulder, tender head of humerus and acromio-clavicular joint.

Review the shoulder radiographs first, then assess the acromio-clavicular joint radiographs on the next page.

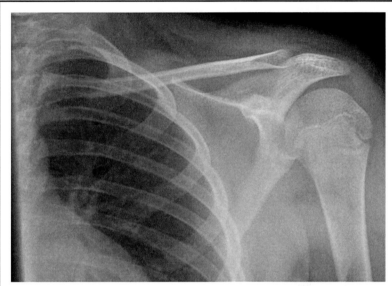

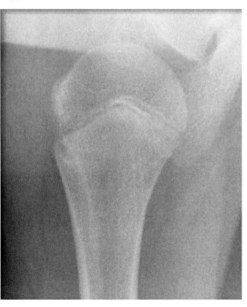

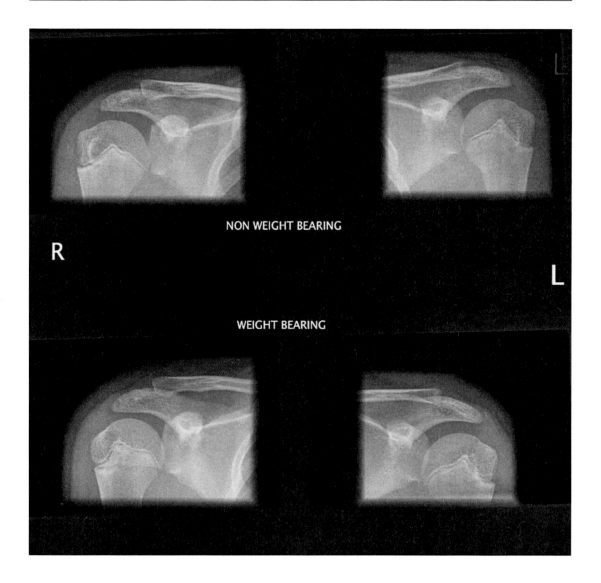

NON WEIGHT BEARING

R

L

WEIGHT BEARING

Answer to Case 101

The shoulder radiographs show no bony injury; however the anterior posterior radiograph is of poor quality, and the arm is internally rotated instead of externally rotated, possibly masking some pathology.

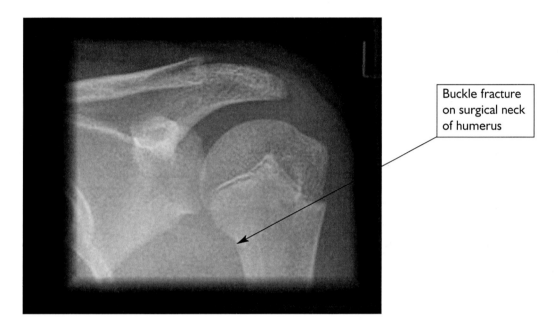

Buckle fracture on surgical neck of humerus

On reviewing the acromioclavicular joint views, the acromio-clavicular joints are aligned normally (remember to check the alignment of the undersurface of the acromion and clavicle when looking for subluxation). On the second group of radiographs the left arm is in the true anteroposterior position with the arm externally rotated, and demonstrates a buckle fracture of the medial aspect of the surgical neck. This emphasises the importance of obtaining as high a quality radiograph as possible, in order not to miss an injury.

Case 102

Side of face was hit by a falling branch. Now unable to open and close mouth.

Comment on image.

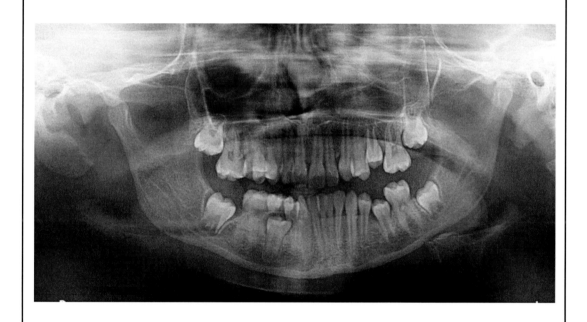

Answer to Case 102

There is dislocation of the right tempero mandible joint.

Case 103

Patient fell from wall injuring their ankle.

Describe the radiographs.

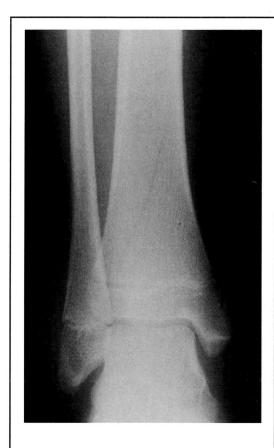

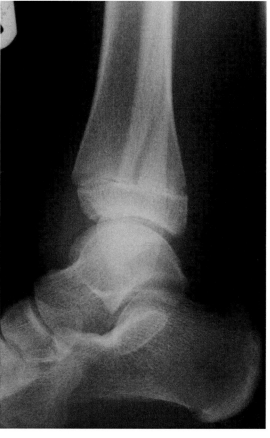

Answer to Case 103

There is a Salter Harris type II injury of the distal tibia. The lateral view demonstrates the malalignment of the anterior tibia metaphysis and anterior tibia epiphysis, clearly demonstrating that the physeal plate is involved in the injury.

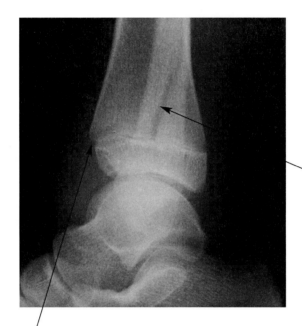

Fracture line is in tibia, as it stops at tibial physeal plate. Fibula physeal plate is more distal.

Malalignment of tibia epiphysis and metaphysis demonstrating disruption of the physeal plate

Case 104

Patient fell from trampoline, now painful ankle.

Describe the radiographs.

Would any other radiographic views be helpful?

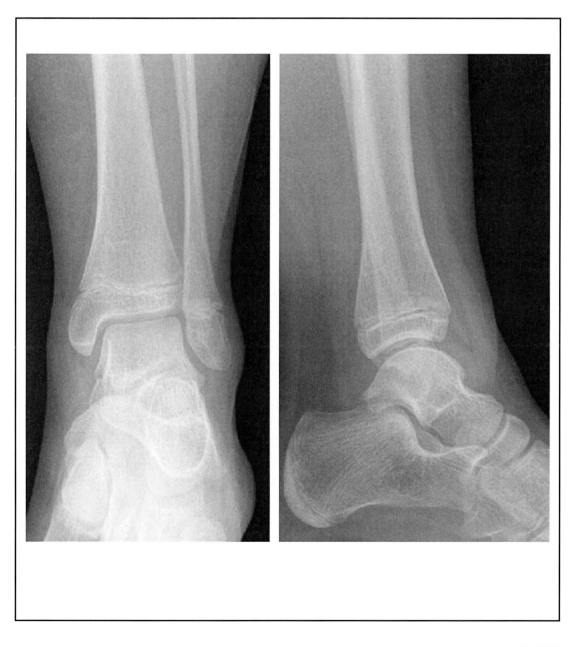

Answer to Case 104

There is a large joint effusion (see short arrows below). There is a fracture of the distal tibia metaphysis which appears to stop at the tibial physeal plate. There is malalignment of the tibial metaphysis and epiphysis indicating disruption of the physeal plate (within the circled area). This appears to be a Salter Harris II of the distal tibia as in Case 103, although a little more subtle. On closer inspection there appears to be widening of the tibial physeal plate laterally and a hint of a lucent line through the epiphysis. An oblique view is required to rule out a triplane fracture.

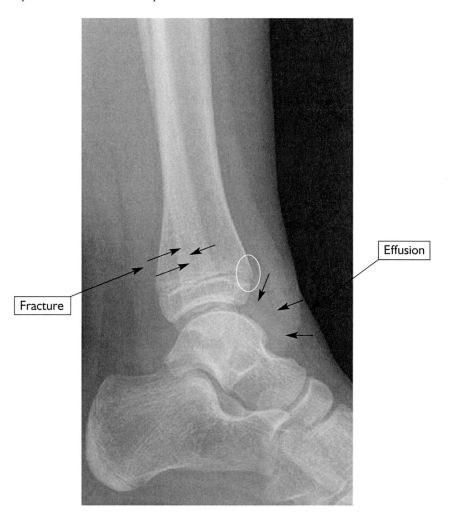

Fracture

Effusion

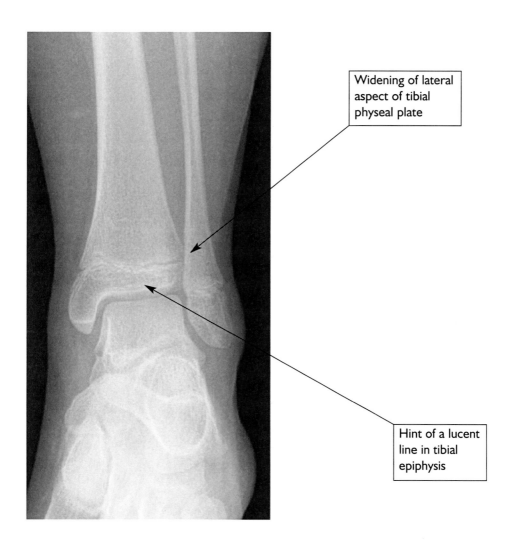

Widening of lateral aspect of tibial physeal plate

Hint of a lucent line in tibial epiphysis

309

The oblique view below clearly demonstrates a fracture through the epiphysis. This is a two-part triplane fracture (Figure 11.1) which requires different management to a Salter Harris II fracture of the distal tibia. See Case 51.

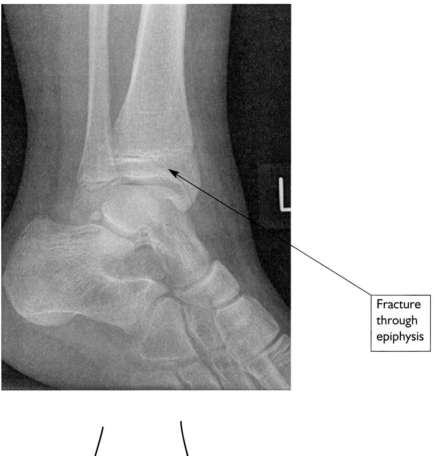

Fracture
through
epiphysis

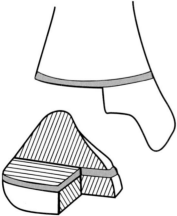

figure 11.1
Two-part juvenile triplane fracture

Case 105

Patient fell from bicycle, injuring knee.

Describe the radiographs.

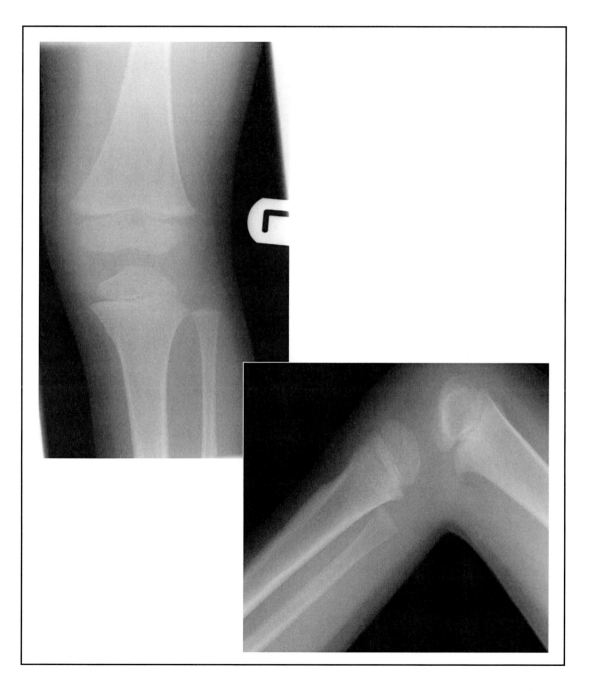

Answer to Case 105

There is a subtle buckle fracture of the medial aspect of the proximal tibial metaphysis. The indentation on the superior aspect of the proximal tibia is normal and is the area where the tibial tuberosity will form.

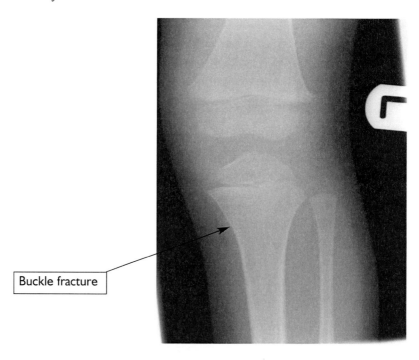

Buckle fracture

Normal tibial indentation, where tibial tuberosity will form

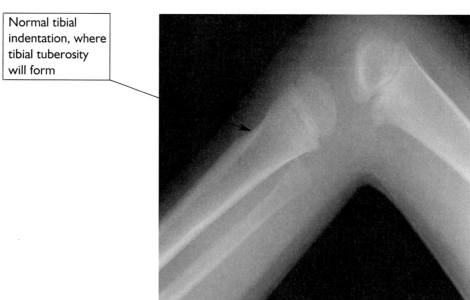

Case 106

Patient fell on outstretched hand. Now has a painful forearm, unable to move.

Describe radiographs.

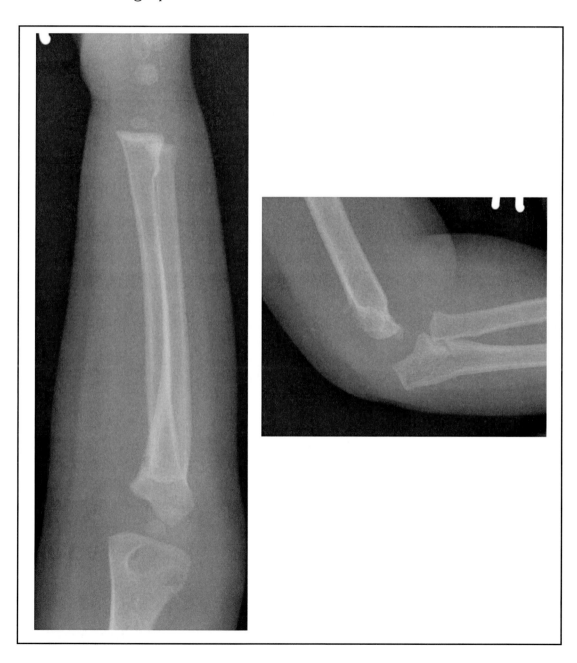

Answer to Case 106

The forearm radiograph demonstrates a torus fracture of the dorsal aspect of the distal radius, with slight dorsal angulation of the distal part (remember the distal radius is normally angulated 10 to 15 degrees volarly). If you review the elbow on the same radiograph there is a break in the cortex of the distal humerus lateral aspect. Following this, a lateral elbow radiograph was taken; this not only demonstrates a joint effusion (positive anterior and posterior fat pads) and supracondylar fracture, but also a fracture of the proximal olecranon.

Case 107

Patient hyper-extended fingers during games. Now has a painful little finger metacarpal.

Describe the radiographs.

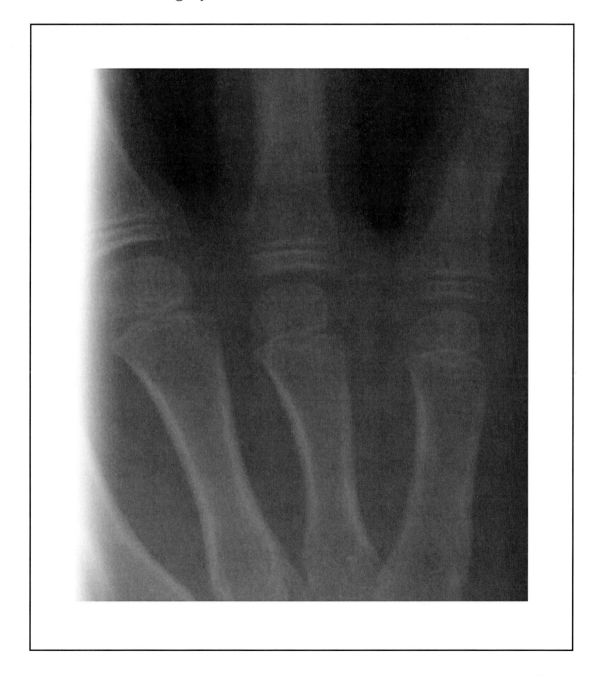

Answer to Case 107

There is a Salter Harris type II fracture of the proximal phalanx of the little finger, ulnar aspect.

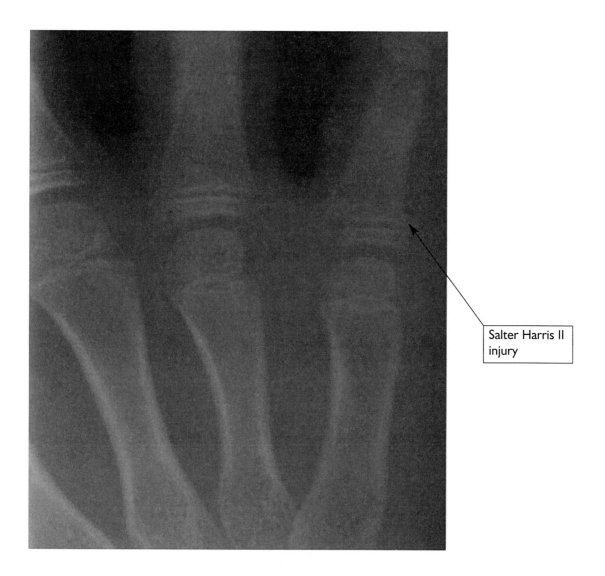

Salter Harris II
injury

Case 108

Adolescent fell during football training, injuring ankle.

Describe the radiographs.

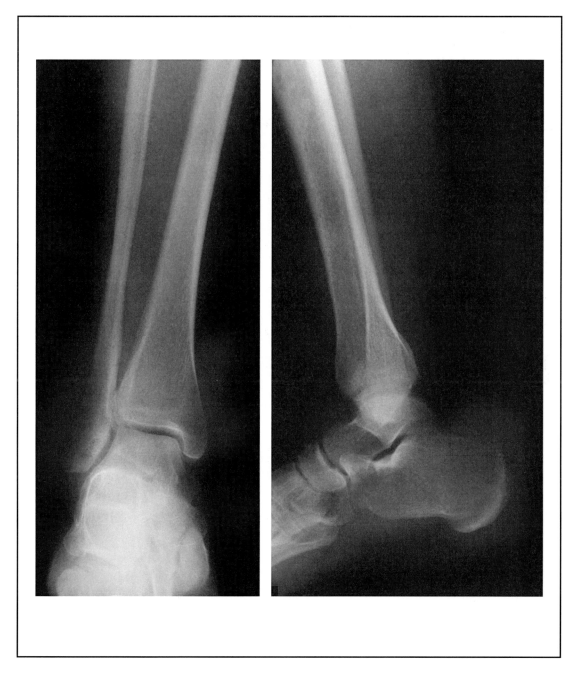

Answer to Case 108

There is a juvenile Tillaux fracture. A careful look at the peroneal groove demonstrates a step in the cortex and a lucent line in the distal lateral tibia. The fracture is also demonstrated on the lateral view anterior to the distal fibula (see Case 51).

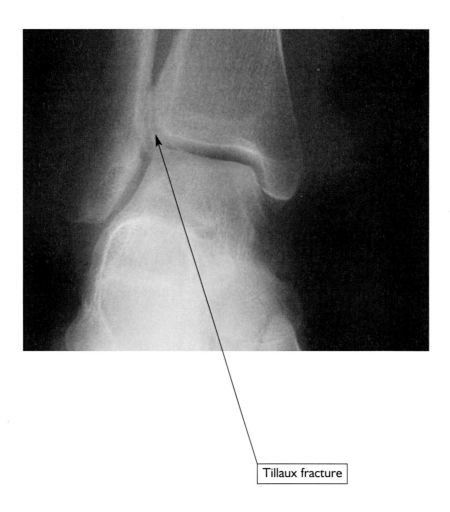

Tillaux fracture

Case 109

Patient plays cricket frequently, is suffering from pain and stiffness in elbow and has restricted movement.

Describe the radiographs.

What is the name for this condition?

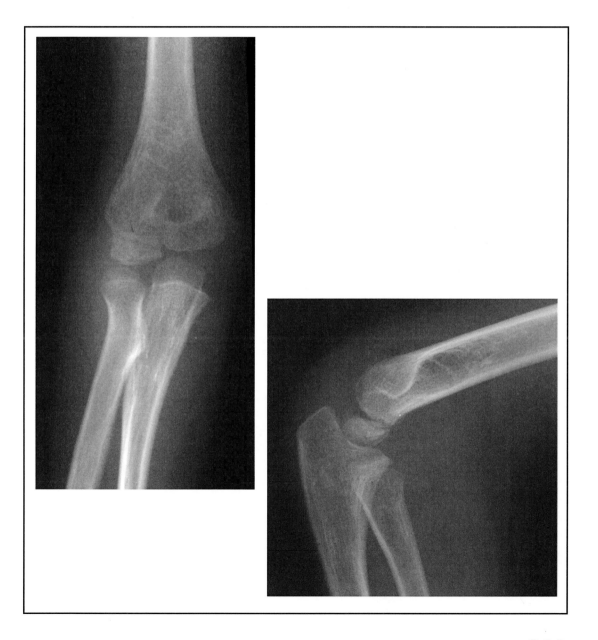

Answer to Case 109

There is a joint effusion (positive posterior and anterior fat pads). The cortex of the capitellum is irregular, with subarticular lucency and small sclerotic area. This is Panner's disease, avascular necrosis of the capitellum, sometimes called 'little leaguer's elbow', because of its frequency in young baseball players. Normally occurs in males between 5 and 10 years of age. Clinically the patient has pain and stiffness, with restricted range of movement. The radiograph may demonstrate joint effusion, sclerosis, fragmentation and decreased size of the capitellum.

Another case of Panner's disease with more fragmentation of the capitellum is demonstrated below.

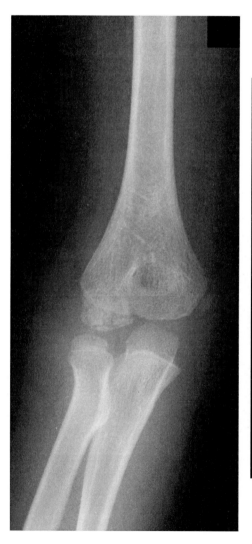
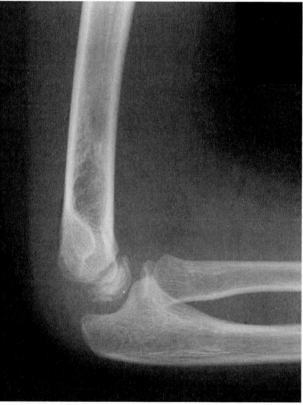

Case 110

Patient fell from tree, now painful forearm.

Describe the radiographs.

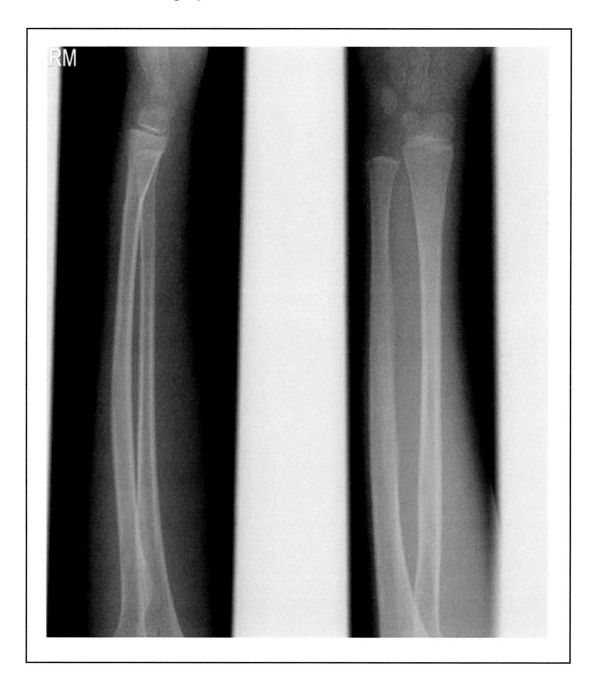

Answer to Case 110

There is a subtle torus fracture of the distal radius, with some increase in volar angulation of the distal radius.

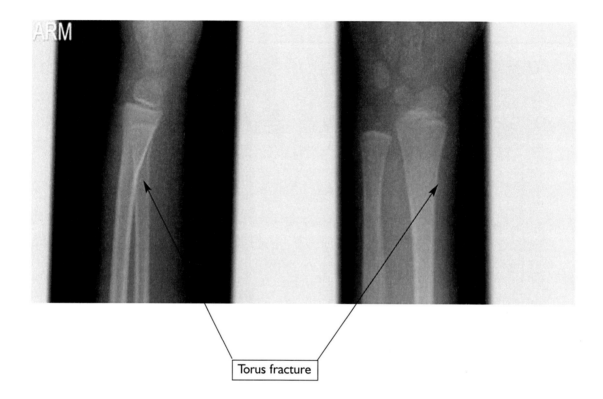

Torus fracture

Case 111

Adolescent fell onto outstretched hand, now bony tenderness in scaphoid.

Describe the radiographs.

What is the main complication with scaphoid injuries?

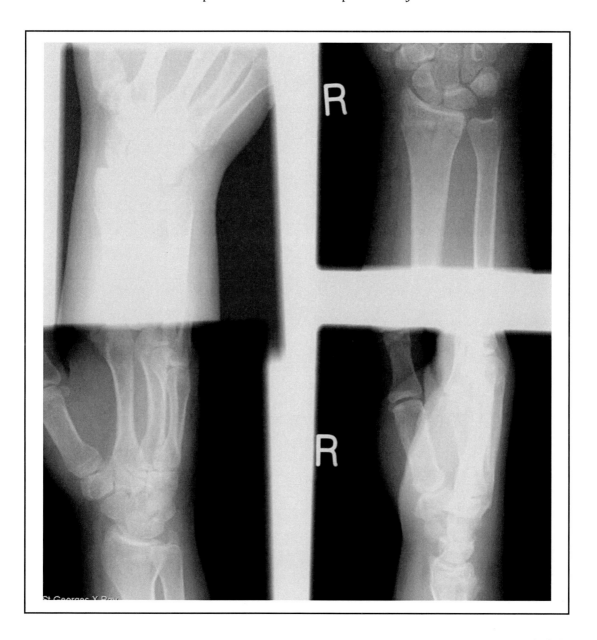

Answer to Case 111

There is a transverse fracture of the distal radius (at the level of the closing physeal plate), with a second longitudinal fracture line. The lateral radiograph shows dorsal angulation of the distal radius. Although the Stetcher's view is too underpenetrated to be diagnostic, the other radiographic views do not demonstrate a scaphoid fracture. Scaphoid fractures and carpal injuries are rare under 12 years of age (see Case 1).

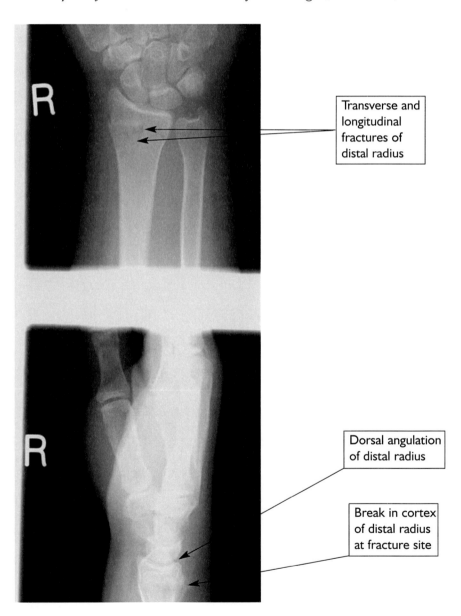

Transverse and longitudinal fractures of distal radius

Dorsal angulation of distal radius

Break in cortex of distal radius at fracture site

The scaphoid has two blood supplies, one at the distal pole, the other at the waist of the scaphoid; the supply at the waist is a development or continuation of a division of the radial artery that also supplies the distal pole. Most fractures occur at the waist of the scaphoid. A fracture at the waist of the scaphoid may affect the blood supply at the waist resulting in avascular necrosis of the proximal pole of the scaphoid. A fracture of the distal pole of the scaphoid will not result in avascular necrosis – as the distal fragment will receive its blood supply from the distal blood vessels, whilst those entering at the waist will supply the rest of the scaphoid. Fractures of the proximal pole of the scaphoid will result in avascular necrosis of the proximal fracture as it is cut off from its blood supply at the waist and distally. Scaphoid fractures are at risk from delayed union, non-union and avascular necrosis of the proximal pole.

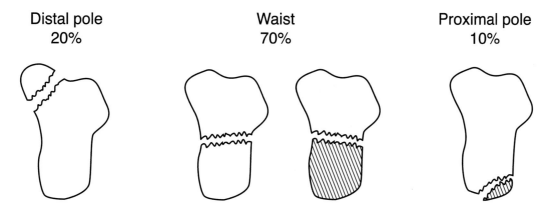

Figure 11.2

Scaphoid fractures – shaded areas highlight areas at risk from avascular necrosis following fracture

Below is another patient with non-union of the scaphoid and avascular necrosis following fracture.

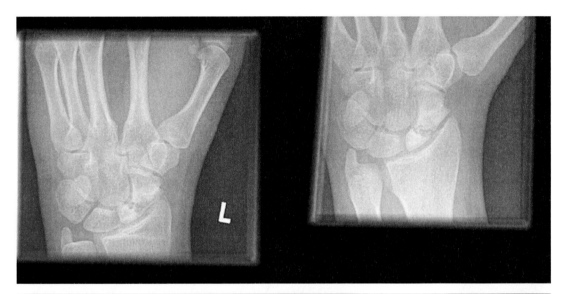

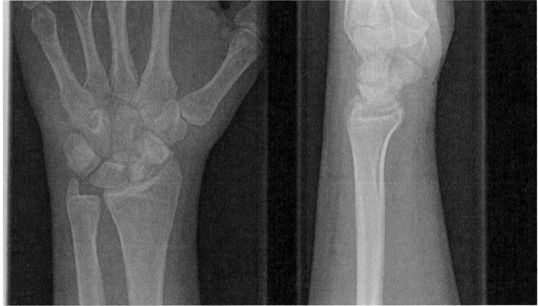

Case 112

Patient hit a wall.

Describe the radiographs.

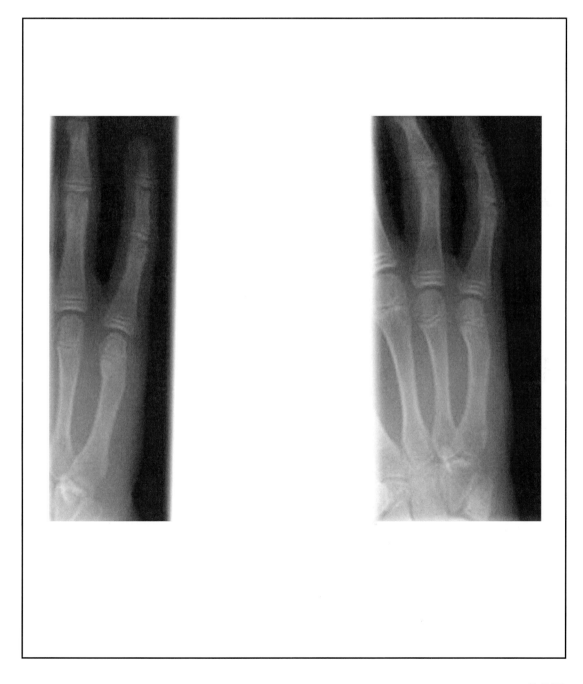

Answer to Case 112

There is a greenstick fracture (notice break in cortex volar aspect) of the distal part of the fifth metacarpal (little finger metacarpal), with some volar angulation of the distal part. It is a typical injury following a direct blow with the clenched fist.

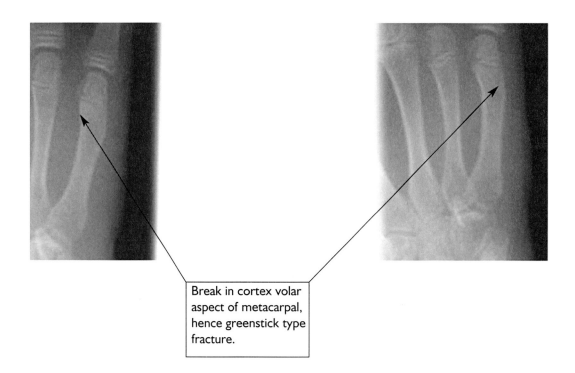

Break in cortex volar aspect of metacarpal, hence greenstick type fracture.

Case 113

Patient fell from bike, injuring knee.

Describe the radiographs.

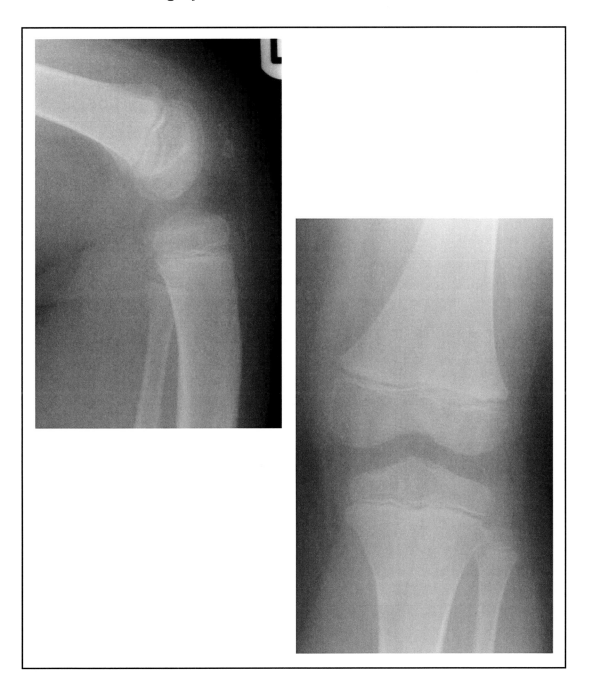

Answer to Case 113

There is no bony injury. The bifid patella is a normal development variant and not a fracture, which will continue to form a bipartite patella.

Case 114

Patient fell onto outstretched hand, now bony tenderness of distal radius.

Describe the radiographs.

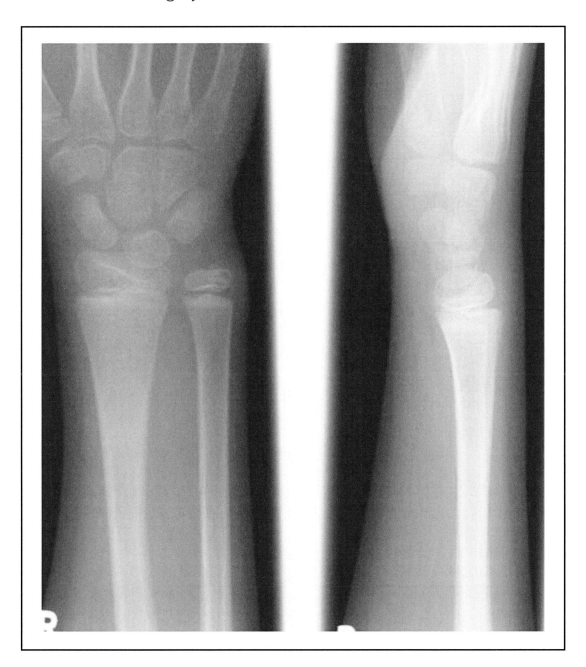

Answer to Case 114

There is a subtle buckle fracture of the distal radius, ulnar aspect, which coincides with the site of bony tenderness.

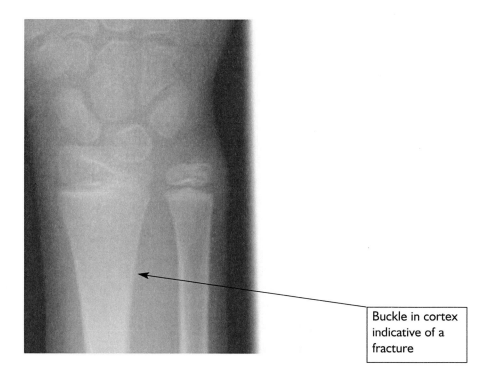

Buckle in cortex indicative of a fracture

Case 115

Patient fell, inverting foot.

Describe the radiographs.

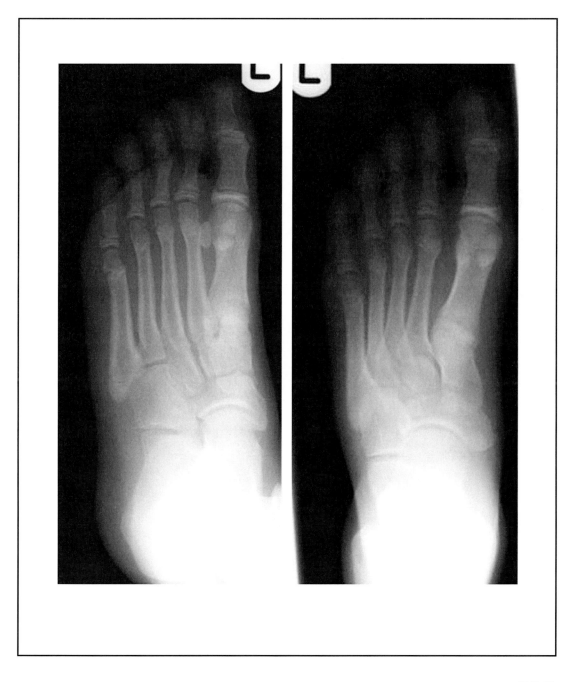

Answer to Case 115

There is a transverse fracture of the base of the fifth metatarsal (see Cases 54 and 55) with associated soft tissue swelling.

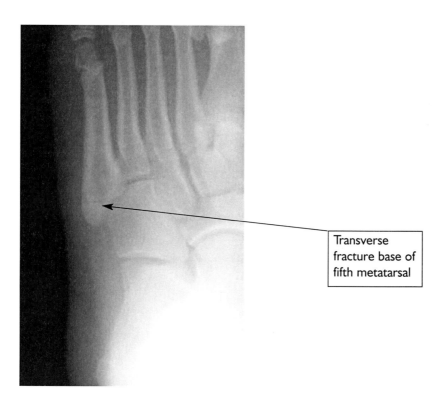

Transverse fracture base of fifth metatarsal

Case 116

Patient fell off pushbike, injuring elbow, all movements painful.

Write a provisional image evaluation.

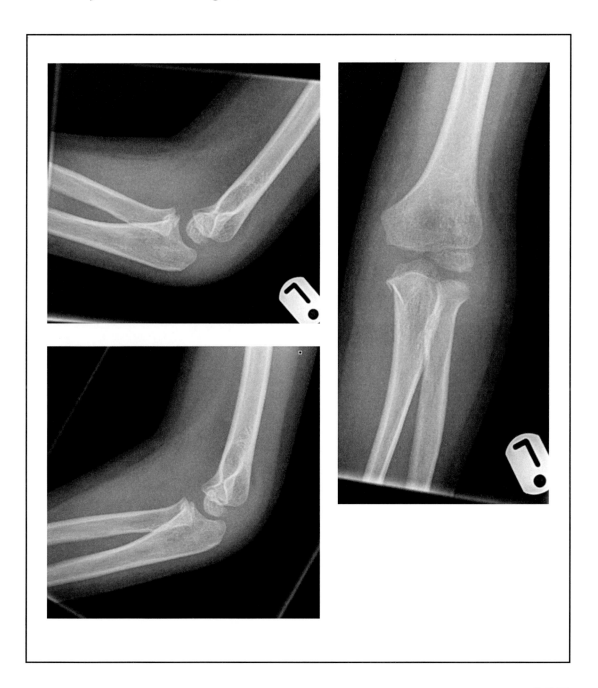

Answer to Case 116

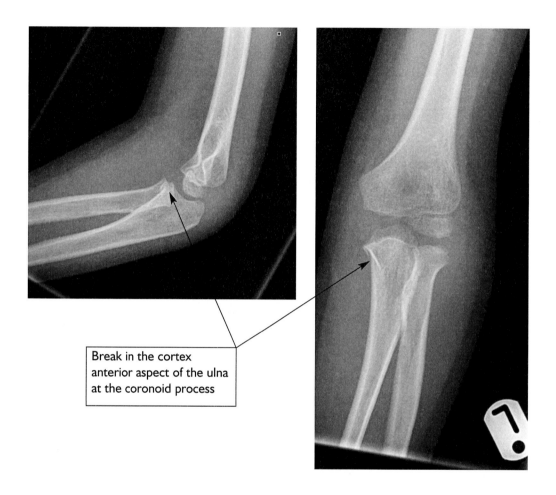

Break in the cortex anterior aspect of the ulna at the coronoid process

The lateral view demonstrates, as we have seen previously, a joint effusion – in this case, positive anterior and posterior fat pads, being indicative of fracture. There is a fracture of the coronoid process. Coronoid process fractures are sometimes seen when there is a dislocation at the elbow joint, but not in this case.

Case 117

Painful ankle, following fall from bicycle.

Comment on the images. What may happen next?

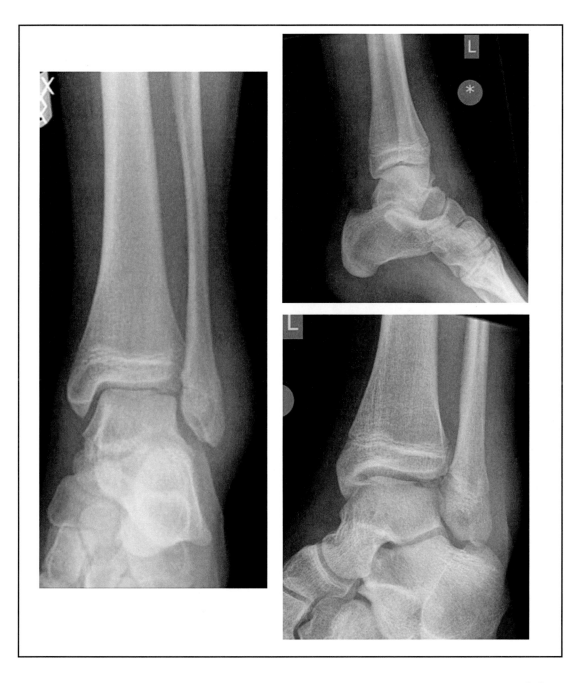

Answer to Case 117

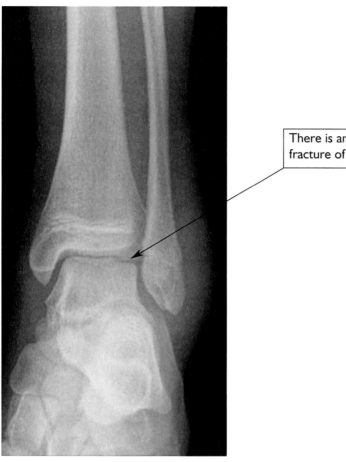

There is an osteochondral fracture of the talar dome

There is an osteochondral fracture of the talar dome, normally caused by a tangential force. These are commonly found at relatively rounded surfaces, such as the talar dome, femoral condyles and sometimes the capitellum. The problem with osteochondral fractures is that only the bony component of the injury (the 'osteo') is demonstrated on radiographs. The cartilage component (the'chondral'), which may be larger than the bony component, is not visualised radiographically.

All these injuries therefore require an MRI scan in order to demonstrate the full extent of the injury. An osteochondral fracture, which may look extremely small and insignificant on a radiograph, may on MRI be seen to involve a significantly large amount of cartilage. Hence it is important that the image reviewer not only sees the osteochondral fracture but recognises its significance, so that the correct pathway is activated.

Case 118

Fell from shed roof, injuring ankle. Unable to weight bear.

Describe the injuries.

Should any further radiographs be considered?

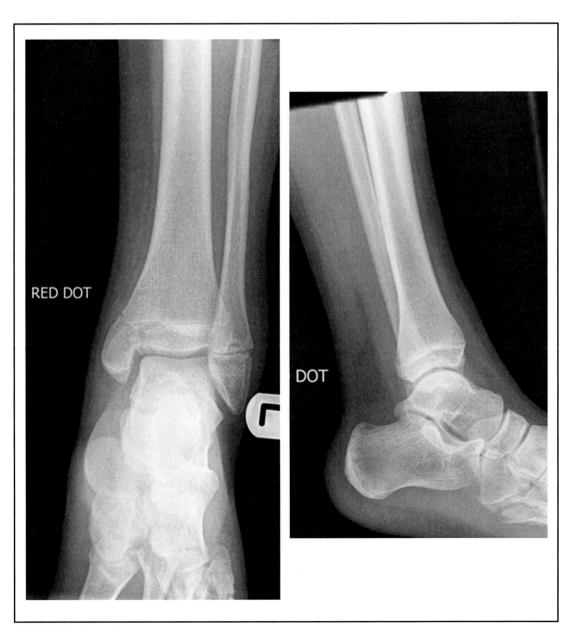

Answer to Case 118

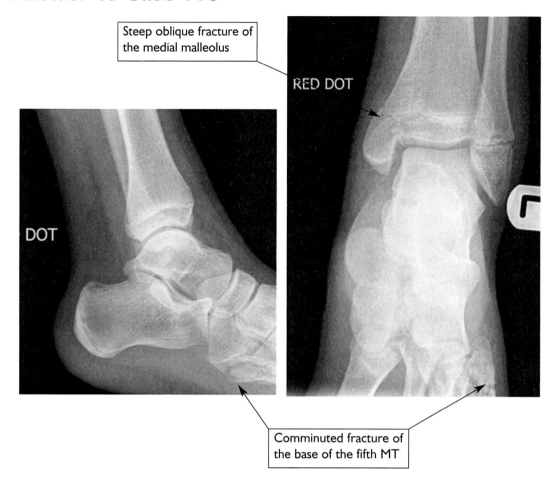

Steep oblique fracture of the medial malleolus

RED DOT

DOT

Comminuted fracture of the base of the fifth MT

Firstly there is a comminuted fracture of the base of the fifth metatarsal, which highlights the fact that you should carefully review all areas of the x-ray image to ensure that an unsuspected injury or pathology is not missed. Foot x-rays should be carried out to assess this injury further and assess for other fractures of the foot. It is a significant injury that will have required a moderate force to occur, so there may be other unsuspected fractures of the foot.

The ankle demonstrates a steep oblique fracture of the medial malleolus, but no fracture of the distal fibula. A proximal fibula fracture (a so-called high fibula fracture) needs to be ruled out, with full-length tibia and fibula x-rays. The reason for this is that if a high fibula fracture is present, as well as the medial malleolus fracture, then it becomes an unstable ankle injury, which affects the way the patient is managed (the so-called Maisonneuve type fracture). With this type of injury, the patient often has no pain proximally, all the pain being distal around the ankle joint.

Lauge Hausen classified injuries of the ankle, dividing them into four mechanisms of injury. The high fibula fracture was a result of a pronation lateral rotation injury. He described each of the four mechanisms of injury using a staging mechanism. With the high fibula fracture, the first stage is a fracture of the medial malleolus or injury of the deltoid ligament, the second stage is injury of the anterio distal tibio-fibula ligament, and the third stage is the interosseous membrane being disrupted from the level of the ankle joint to the level of the high fibula fracture. A high fibula fracture then occurs above the syndesmosis; and the fourth stage is a fracture of the posterior medial malleolus or posterior distal tibia fibula ligament. If the injury is at the fourth stage, there is nothing holding the tibia and fibula together from the ankle joint to the high fibula fracture, which means that it is a highly unstable injury. This is why it is important to identify this injury, as it significantly alters patient management and would require surgery.

In this case, no high fibula fracture was identified on further images.

Case 119

Patient fell, injuring ankle.

Is there an injury?

Describe the radiographs.

Do these images give rise to any pathological concern?

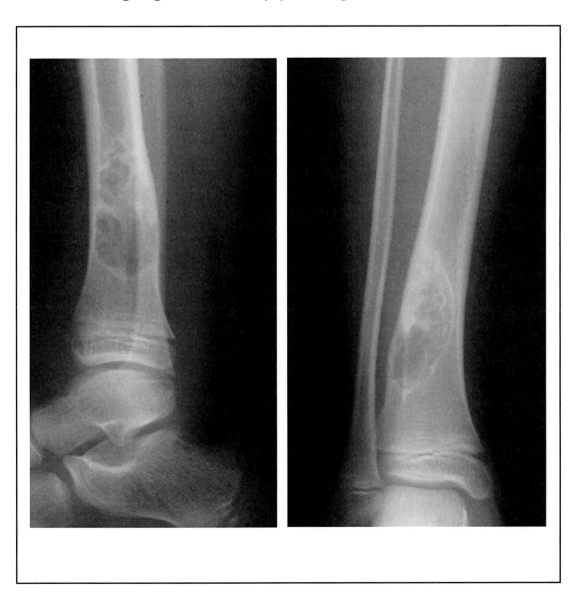

Answer to Case 119

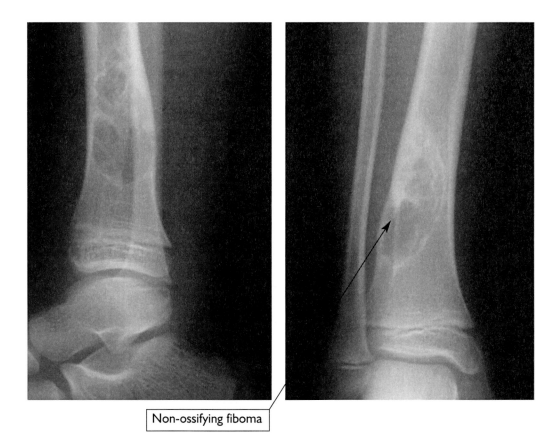

Non-ossifying fiboma

There is no fracture present. There is a well-defined (with some sclerotic borders), slightly expansile lytic lesion in the diaphysis of the distal tibia. This is a non-ossifying fibroma, a benign lesion, one of the so-called 'leave me alone lesions'. It is probably one of the most common benign lesions. It is identical to a fibrous cortical defect; non-ossifying fibromas being identified as larger than 2 cm, whereas fibrous cortical defects are smaller than 2 cm.

Both are normally asymptomatic, unless they are fractured; they generally occur in the metaphysis and are intracortical. Non-osssifying fibromas, in particular, tend to be lobulated, with a so-called soap bubble appearance. Both tend to have an overall oval appearance and align with the long axis of the bone. Both are to be found in patients under the age of 30 years. In a narrow bone, such as the fibula, the lesion may appear to involve the whole diameter of the bone.

Case 120

In goal, fell trying to save ball, hyperextending arm. Now unable to lower humerus to side of body.

What is the injury?

How does it occur?

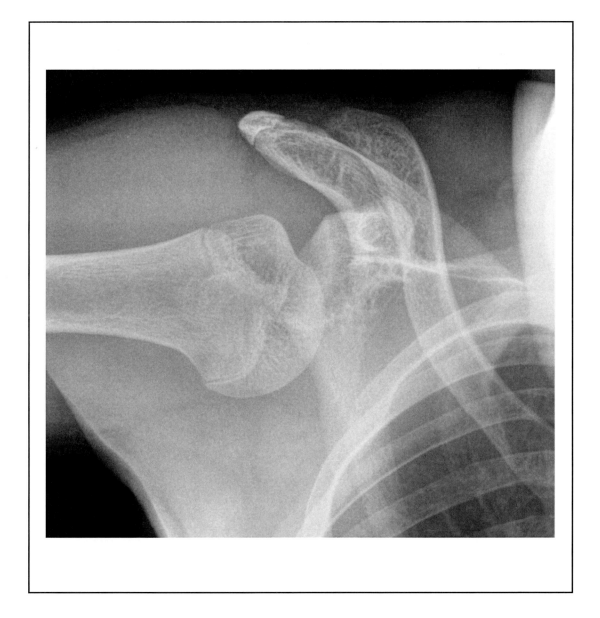

Answer to Case 120

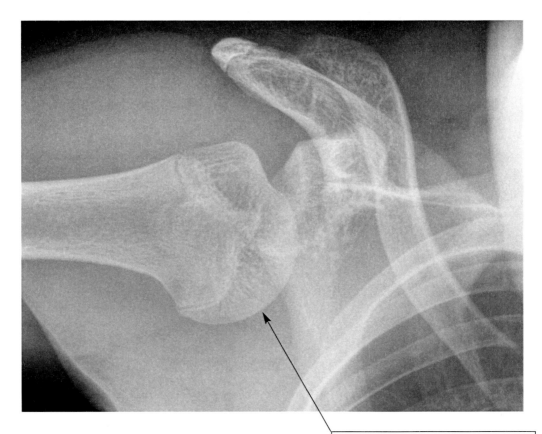

Articular surface of humeral head is pointing inferiorly; it is not articulating with the glenoid; hence inferior dislocation – luxatio erecta

The articular surface of the humeral head is pointing inferiorly; it is no longer articulating with the glenoid; hence it is an inferior dislocation, the so-called luxatio erecta. This occurs as the arm is hyperabducted, resulting in the humeral head hitting the acromion and being levered away from the glenoid, leading to an inferior dislocation. The patient normally presents with the arm extended and the hand resting on the head. This occurs more commonly in adults, although it is not as common as an anterior or posterior dislocation of the gleno-humeral joint.

Case 121

Patella subluxed/dislocated whilst running, then relocated, now difficulty weight bearing.

Write a provisional image evaluation.

What additional view should be done if possible when reviewing a suspected dislocated patella?

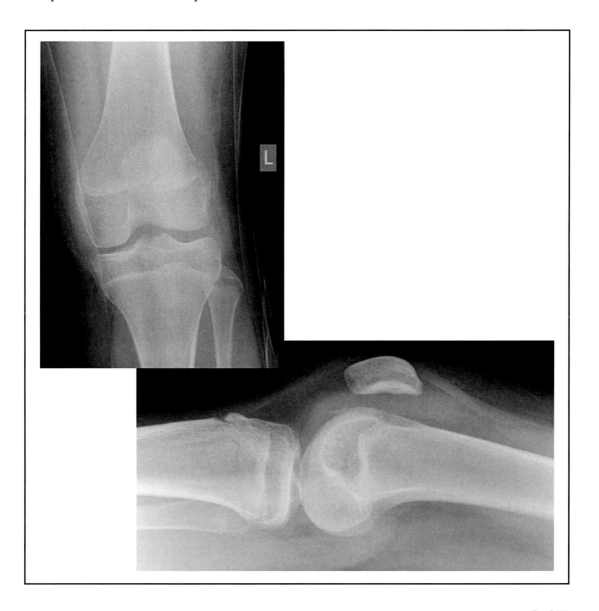

Answer to Case 121

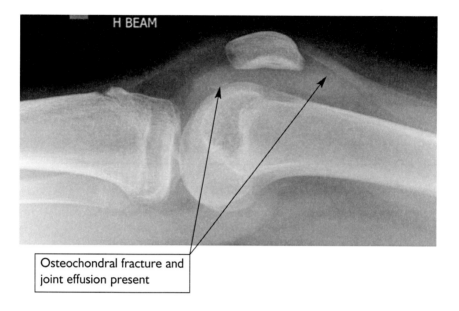

H BEAM

Osteochondral fracture and joint effusion present

There is a moderate joint effusion and an osteochondral fracture. As previously discussed, osteochondral fractures should all have an MRI to assess how much cartilage is involved. When the patella dislocates, it can result in an osteochondral fracture from the femoral condyles, due to the tangential force it produces as it dislocates. When reviewing a query dislocated patella, a skyline view should be done as well, to rule out or confirm remaining dislocation; it may also help with the search for osteochondral fractures. The reviewer should also assess for patella alta, as it is strongly associated with recurring patella dislocation.

Case 122

Fell onto shoulder, now painful.

Write a provisional image evaluation.

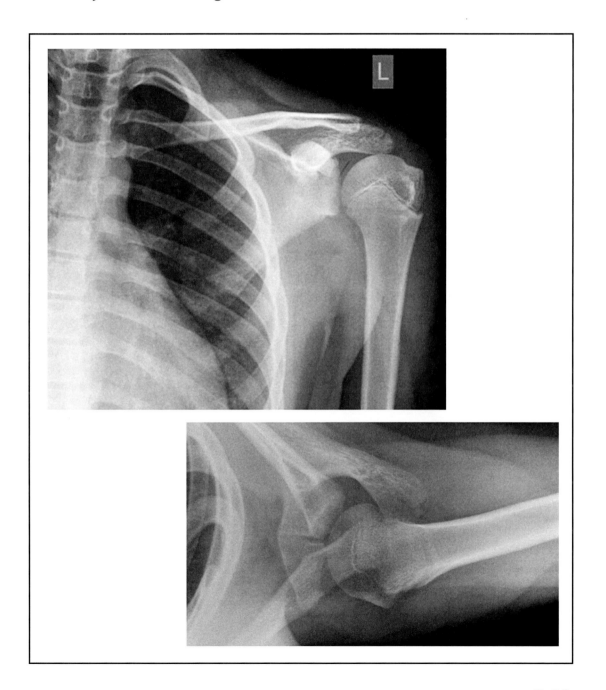

Answer to Case 122

There is no bony injury and no dislocation. The adolescent shoulder has several apophysis, acromion and coracoid (see Case 45), and the glenoid is made from tri-radiate cartilage. The image reviewer has to be careful not to mistake any of these normal growth appearances for fractures.

Case 123

Patient hit a wall with hand, now painful.

Write a provisional image evaluation.

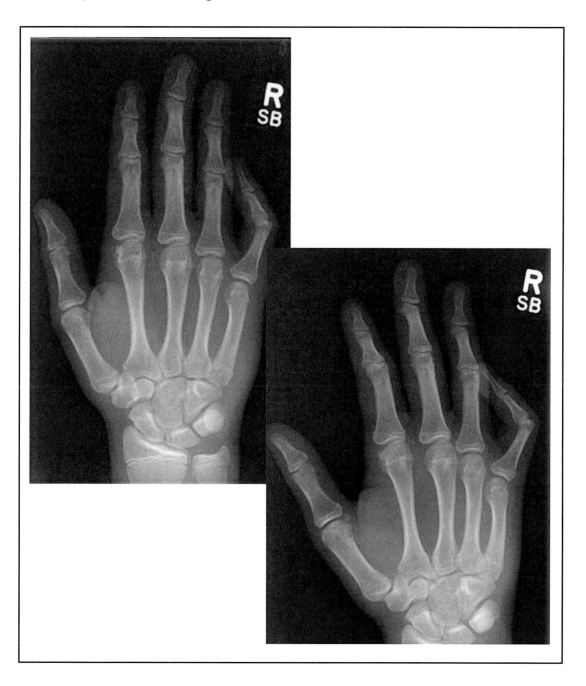

Answer to Case 123

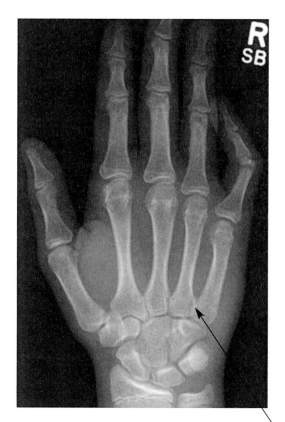 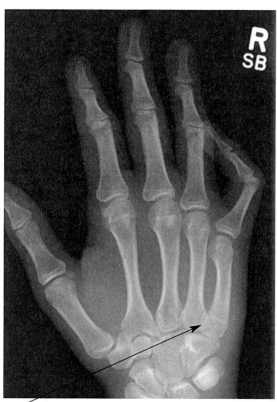

There is a break in the cortex and transverse lucent line at the base of the little finger metacarpal: hence a minimally displaced transverse fracture of the base of the little finger metacarpal

There is a break in the cortex and transverse lucent line at the base of the little finger metacarpal: hence a minimally displaced transverse fracture. However, the reviewer has to be careful that normal physeal lines are not mistaken for fractures and vice versa.

The proximal interphalangeal joint of the little finger appears subluxed, but it is probably projectional. If there is any clinical concern at this area then dedicated finger views are required.

Case 124

Child awoke, unable to stand on heel.

Write a provisional image evaluation.

Would any other view be helpful?

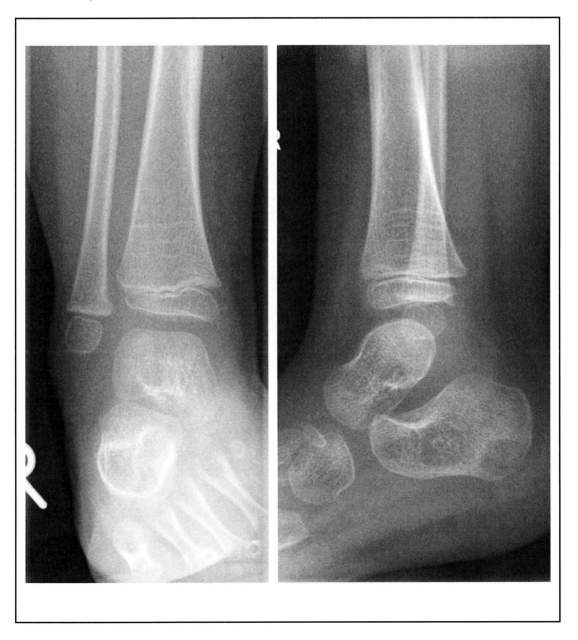

Answer to Case 124

There is a well-defined lucent area plantar aspect of the calcaneum. The radiographer did an additional calcaneal view, which demonstrated complete loss of the calcaneal cortex. This is osteomyelitis. In this age group, the most likely cause is staphylococcus aureus; and at this site it is most likely that the child stood on something that broke the skin and set up an infective process.

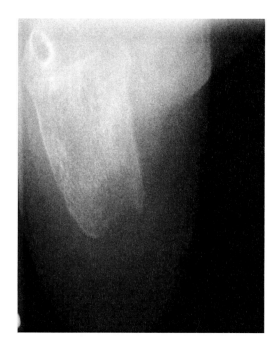

Staphylococcus aureus is the most common organism that causes osteomyelitis in children (and adults). However, in neonates group B streptococcus is a more common cause. In children the blood vessels in the metaphysis tend to occur in loops, in which the blood flow can be quite sluggish. There is also a lack of phagocytes in the metaphysis region. Hence the metaphysis region in children can be prone to osteomyelitis. In infants the metaphyseal vessels anastomose with the epiphyseal vessels. If there is an infection in the metaphysis, it may therefore cross over to the epiphysis and involve the joint and possibly lead to slipped epiphysis. In the child the metaphyseal vessels do not anastomose with epiphyseal vessels so an infection in the metaphysis will not affect the epiphysis.

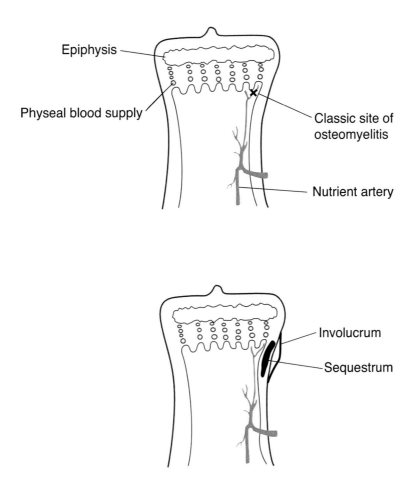

Figure 11.1 **Pathogenesis of long bone osteomyelitis**

If the infection continues, the periosteum tries to seal off the infection by wrapping itself around the infected cortex; this is called the involucrum. Beneath the involucrum, the cortex may die and become sclerotic in appearance on the radiograph; this is called the sequestrum. If the infection continues to progress, channels (called lacunae) will form and these take the pus to the surface.

To conclude, if you see a lucent area in the metaphysis of a child, be highly suspicious of osteomyelitis.

Case 125

This adult patient noticed a lump in their left groin. In his youth, the patient was keen on sport.

What injury may the patient have had in adolescence?

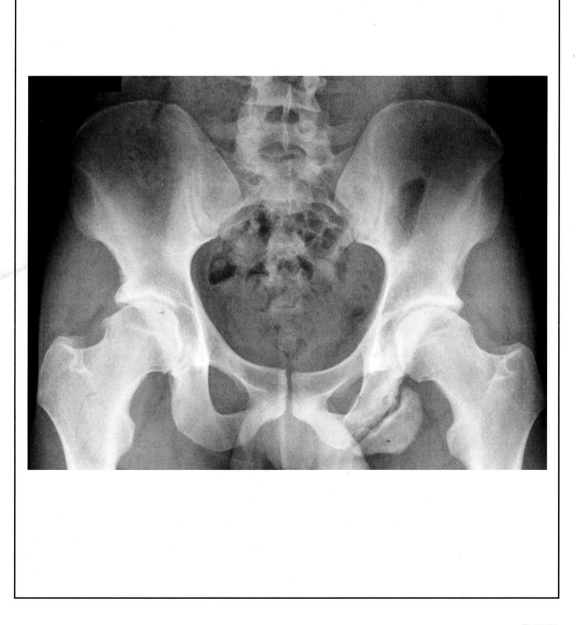

Answer to Case 125

There is an old avulsion of the apophysis of the ischial tuberoscity, where the hamstrings attach. Avulsions of the pelvic apophysis are common between 12 and 17 years of age, as the apophysis is weaker than the attached muscle; and they are associated with sporting activity. These pelvic avulsions are common in sprinters, long jumpers and hurdlers. If the injury in this case occurred in an adult, it would result in a ruptured hamstring.

These avulsions of the pelvis have a tendency to repair themselves with substantial bone being deposited, with they result that they are sometimes mistaken for infections or tumours. Hence it is imperative in these cases to obtain a detailed history from the patient (see Case 79).

Reading List/Bibliography

Annals of the ICRP (1996). *Use of Ionising Radiation and its Application in Diagnostic Imaging*: London: ICRP.

Bhatia, N.N., Pirpiris, M. and Otsuka, N.Y. (1995). Body mass index in patients with slipped capital femoral epiphysis. *Journal of Paediatric Orthopaedics*. 15, 349–56

Borden, S. (1975). Roentgen recognition of acute plastic bowing fractures of the forearm in children. in *American Journal of Radiology*. 124, 524.

Burnett, S., and Tyler, A. (2000). *A–Z of Orthopaedic Radiology*. London: W.B. Saunders.

Caffey, J. (1978). *Paediatric X-ray Diagnosis,* 7th edn. London: Year Book Medical Publishers.

Carty, H. (2004). *Imaging Children*, 2nd edn. London: Churchill Livingstone.

Chapman, S. and Nakielny, R. (1995). *Aids to Radiological Differential Diagnosis*, 3rd edn. London: W.B. Saunders.

Crandall, W.V. and Langer, J.C. (1999). Primary omental torsion presenting as hip pain and limp. *Journal of Pediatric Gastroenterology and Nutrition*. 28, 95–96.

Crowe, J.E. and Swischuk, L.E. (1977). Acute bowing fractures of the forearm in children: A frequently missed injury. in *American Journal of Radiology* 128, 981.

Dandy, D.J. and Edwards, D.J. (1998). *Essentials of Orthopaedics and Trauma*, 3rd edn. London: Churchill Livingstone.

Greenspan, A. and Gershwin, M.E. (1990). *Radiology of the Arthrides – a Clinical Approach*. London, New York: JB Lippincott, Gower Medical Publishing.

Helms, Clyde A. (1995). *Fundamentals of Skeletal Radiology*, 2nd edn. London: W.B. Saunders.

Kalliola, S. and Vuopio-Varkila, J. (1999). Neonatal group B streptococcal disease in Finland: a ten-year nationwide study. *The Pediatric Infectious Disease Journal*. 18, 806–10.

Kastrissianakis, K. and Beattie, T.F. (2010). Transient synovitis of the hip; more evidence for a viral aetiology. *European Journal of Medicine*.
http://www.ncbi.nlm.nih.gov/pubmed/20523221 (last accessed 11.10.2015)

Keats, T. (2001). *Atlas of Normal Roentgen Variants that may Simulate Disease*, 7th edn. London: Mosby

Landin, L.A. (1983). Children's ankle fractures: classification and epidemiology. *Acta Orthopaedica Scandinavica* 54, 634–40.

Lehmann, C.L., Arons, R.R., Loder, R.T. and Vitale, M.G. (2006). The epidemiology of slipped capital femoral epiphysis: an update. *Journal of Paediatric Orthopaedics*. 26, 286–90.

Loder, R.T., Schwartz, E.M. and Hesenger, R.N. (1993). Behavioural characteristics of children with Legg–Calve–Perthes disease. *Journal of Paediatric Orthopaedics*. 13, 598–601.

Manaster, B.J. (1989). *Handbooks in Radiology; Skeletal Radiology*. London:Year Book Medical Publishers.

NICE (2003). Updated September 2007. *Managing Head Injury: NICE Guidelines*. London: National Institute for Health and Care Excellence.

NICE (2014). *NICE Clinical Guidelines 176. Head injury: Triage, assessment, investigation and early management of head injury in children, young people and adults*. London: National Institute for Health and Care Excellence.

Nicholson, D.A. and Driscoll, P.A. (1995) *ABC of Emergency Radiology*. London: W.B. Saunders.

Ozonoff, M.B. (1979). *Paediatric Orthopaediac Radiology*. Philadelphia: W.B. Saunders.

Pang, D. and Wilerger, J.E. (1982). Spinal cord injury without radiographic abnormalities in children. *Journal of Neurosurgery* 57; 114–29.

Perry, D. and Bruce, C. (2010). Evaluating the child who presents with an acute limp. *British Medical Journal.* **341**, c4250.

Raby, N. and de Lacey, G., (2005). *Accident and Emergency Radiology: A Survival Guide*, 2nd edn. London: Elsevier.

Renton, P. (1998). *Orthopaediac Radiology – Pattern Recognition and Differential Diagnosis*, 2nd edn. London: Martin Dunitz.

Resnick, R. (1989). 'Diagnostic imaging of paediatric skeletal trauma' in *Radiologic Clinics of North America* 27(5), 243–9.

Rogers, L.F. (1992). *Radiology of Skeletal Trauma*, 2nd edn. London: Churchill Livingstone.

Royal College of Radiologists (2003). *Making the Best Use of a Department of Clinical Radiology*, 4th edn. London: RCR.

Salter, R.B. and Harris, W.R. (1963). Injuries involving the epiphyseal plate. *Journal of Bone and Joint Surgery*, **45A**, 587.

Sheafor, D.H., Holder, L.E. and Thompson, D. (1997). Scrotal pathology as cause for hip pain. Diagnostic findings on bone scintigraphy. *Clinical Nuclear Medicine.* **22**, 287–91.

Stoker, D.J. and Tilley, E.A. (1989). *Self Assessment in Radiology and Imaging 4 – Orthopaedics.* London: Wolfe Medical Publications Ltd.

Thornton, A. and Gyll, C. (1999). *Children's Fractures.* London: W.B. Saunders.

Tile, M. (1995). *Fractures of the Pelvis and Acetabulum.* Baltimore: Williams and Wilkins.

Tile, M. and Pennal, G.F. (1980). Pelvic disruption: principles of management. *Clinical Orthopaedics* **151**, 56.

Vijlbrief, A.S., Bruijnzeels, M.A. and van der Wouden, J.C. (1992). Incidence and management of transient synovitis of the hip: a study in Dutch general practice. *British Journal of General Practice.* **42**, 426–28.

Wynne-Davies, R. and Gormley, J. (1978). The aetiology of Perthes disease. Genetic, epidemiological and growth factors in 310 Edinburgh and Glasgow patients. *Journal of Bone and Joint Surgery* (British Volume). **60**, 6–14.

Index

Figures in bold type refer to illustrations

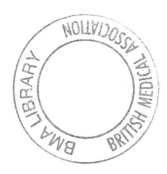